TUTORIALS ON HOMOEOPATHY

Tutorials on Homoeopathy

Donald McD. Foubister
BSc, MB, ChB, DCH, FFHom

BEACONSFIELD PUBLISHERS LTD
Beaconsfield, Bucks, England

First published in 1989

British Library Cataloguing in Publication Data
Foubister, Donald McD. *d. 1988*
    Tutorials on homoeopathy.
    1. Medicine. Homeopathy
    I. Title
    615.5'32

ISBN 0–906584–25–6

Phototypeset by Gem Graphics, Trenance, Mawgan Porth, Cornwall in 10 on 12 point Times.
Printed in Great Britain at The Bath Press, Bath.

To my wife, Agnes Mary

Preface

Donald MacDonald Foubister was born in the town of Kirkwall, the capital of Orkney, on the 31st October 1902. His father was born in the parish of Foubister. His mother, Isabell MacDonald, was born in the Scottish Highlands, where the family usually spent their holidays enjoying the trees and mountains after the bare, treeless, windswept and magical Orkney sea and landscape. Donald had many happy memories of his childhood years, sea bathing and fishing in Scapa Flow, where his own little rowing boat was moored, tempting him to many an escapade of truancy from school. His love of trees and nature led him to decide to study forestry on leaving Kirkwall Grammar School. At the age of seventeen, with this in mind, he entered Aberdeen University, where he obtained a degree in botany, zoology and geology. A family friend suggested he go to Canada for a job in forestry, but on arrival there he found no work available in that line, so he took any job going, often as a farm hand during harvesting. Eventually he became a salesman for a seed company in Nova Scotia, where he worked for five years.

While in Canada he suffered a prolonged back injury from sport activities, which was eventually cured by an osteopath. He found many other sufferers similarly helped, and this gave him an intense interest in the subject and a desire to make it his life's work. He returned to Scotland, where he paid his way through Edinburgh University, gaining his MB, ChB. As a student he happened to be paired in the physiology practical with a fellow student who was brought up in a family of keen homoeopaths. This also interested him and he decided to look further into homoeopathy.

After a few locums in general practice he came to London to pursue his interest in homoeopathy, and in 1937 was appointed house physician at the Royal London Homoeopathic Hospital. During this time he was fortunate in having tuition from Dr Margaret Tyler, Dr Douglas Borland, Sir John Weir and Dr Margery Blackie. During the war he served as a medical officer in England, India and what is now Pakistan, always using homoeopathy despite some official disapproval. He ended his war work 8000 feet up in the Himalayas.

In 1946 he was appointed assistant physician in the Children's Department of the Royal London Homoeopathic Hospital, as well as developing a private practice in London. In 1955 he was admitted as a Fellow in the Faculty of Homoeopathy and in 1956 became consultant homoeopathic physician for diseases of children, among other qualifications. In 1960 he was appointed Dean of the Faculty. He held the Diploma in Child Health of Great Ormond Street Children's Hospital, was consultant physician at the Royal London Homoeopathic Hospital, and on retirement from that hospital was granted honorary consultant status. He was elected President of the Faculty of Homoeopathy 1970–71 and 1971–72. In 1974 he was made an honorary member of the Hahnemann Institute of Brazil. He was made an honorary member of a group of European homoeopathic doctors who held their first congress in Lyons in 1986. During his retirement many doctors from Britain and overseas came to him for tutorials at his home.

Donald discussed and compiled this book with the help of his wife, Agnes, and his stepdaughter, Berenice Benjelloun. He died on the 31st January 1988, as he had lived, with courage.

Contents

Homoeopathy and Paediatrics

Contents

Carcinosin

Other Remedy Pictures

Some Particular Conditions

Contents

Chapter 1

An Introduction

Homoeopathy is defined in Dorland's dictionary as a system of therapeutics founded by Samuel Hahnemann, 1755-1848, in which a disease is treated by drugs which are capable of producing, in health, symptoms of that disease in the patient. These drugs are administered, as homoeopathic remedies, in small doses.

In Hahnemann's day pharmacology, as we know it, did not exist. Information on the drugs used in medical treatment was handed down from one generation to the next, with additions being made by out-standing physicians. Hahnemann, who was recognised throughout Europe as a leading physician and chemist, decided to find out how such drugs acted in health, experimenting on himself, his relatives and doctor colleagues.

He discovered that several drugs produced symptoms similar to those of the diseases for which they had been successfully used. This led to his testing additional drugs not previously used therapeutically, to find out their potential uses as remedies. This study, known as a 'Proving' of the remedy, is still carried on today.

Drugs used in this way can sometimes cause an aggravation in advance of an amelioration. For this reason smaller doses were tried out, leading to the discovery that small doses prepared by dilution and 'succussion', even to the extent that the presence of the drug could no longer be demonstrated by chemical analysis, could be more active than the drug in its crude state. (The process of succussion involves diluting the remedy by stages in an alcohol and water solution, giving it a vigorous mechanical shaking between each stage of dilution.) The products of dilution in this way became known as 'potentised' remedies.

'High' potencies (where this process has been repeated a great many times) can be dangerous in untrained hands. Early this century, Dr James Tyler Kent, one of the leading American homoeopaths, said that he would as soon be in the hands of savages slashing razors as in the hands of an ignorant prescriber of very high potencies.

Some General Considerations

Homoeopathic remedies are prepared in decimal or centesimal potencies. Decimal potencies are prepared by adding one part of the drug to nine parts of pure alcohol, and succussed to ensure even distribution; this is then labelled 1x. One part of 1x diluted in nine parts of alcohol and succussed is labelled 2x, and so on. Centesimal potencies are prepared by adding one part of the drug to ninety-nine of alcohol, and succussed. This is labelled 1c. Further centesimal dilutions are prepared by continuing in the same manner.

Homoeopathy is practised throughout the world, extensively in some places. During the war, when I was serving with the RAF in India, homoeopathic remedies were readily available. I treated malaria with quinine in the usual doses. I treated bacillary dysentery, which in some places was widespread, successfully with homoeopathy, mainly by Pyrogen and Arsenicum Album, each in the 200c potency.

After the war I successfully treated over three hundred cases of primary pneumonia in the children's ward at the Royal London Homoeopathic Hospital; in over eighty per cent with homoeopathy alone, and the remainder with homoeopathy together with penicillin. The homoeopathic approach is to study the individual reaction of the patient, and to choose a remedy which could cover these symptoms plus the symptoms of pneumonia. I used exclusively the 200c potency. This was given every two hours on admission, at whatever stage of the disease. The correctly chosen remedy would be followed by improvement within twelve hours. The dosage was then spread out to every four hours, and later to longer intervals, until cure was evident. By far the most common remedies indicated were Phosphorus or Graphites, in my experience. Occasionally other remedies covered the symptoms, and would be given at the beginning or later if required. Penicillin was given in addition when I considered it necessary.

For some years I treated whooping cough at Shepherds Bush Children's Clinic, as follows. Drosera is the nearest specific, and unless there were definite indications for another remedy, Drosera 30c was given three times a day for four days, then night and morning for a further three days. The children were seen once a week, and Drosera was given at longer intervals. Frequently symptoms of other remedies became apparent, most often Coccus Cacti, the outstanding symptoms of which are morning paroxysmal coughing, ending in vomiting of ropey mucus hanging in long strings from the mouth, or Kali Carb., which covers aggravation at night, especially at 3 a.m., associated with oedema between the upper eyelids and eyebrows, often with a generally puffy face. Whooping cough may occasionally continue for months, and in such cases Drosera 200c, three doses every twelve hours, will clear it up. Another remedy in such cases is Carcinosin 30c, provided that it is otherwise indicated.

The after-effects of injury have been successfully treated for generations. In World War Two the German armed forces were supplied with Arnica Montana 30c in tablet form, to be taken if wounded or otherwise injured, to relieve pain and shock.

Injury remedies have long been used pre- and post-operatively. Six operations of tonsils and/or adenoids were performed weekly in the children's ward of the Royal London Homoeopathic Hospital, including many sent from other regions. My predecessor in charge of the Children's Department, who had had his own tonsils removed, gave routinely before and after these operations Arnica 30c combined with Rhus Tox. 30c, and I continued in this way. Rhus Tox. covers pain on first movement followed later by relief. Children who were obviously worried were given one dose of Phosphorus 30c. This remedy is also useful for anxiety before a visit to the dentist. Rhus Tox. 30c is also usually effective for a sprained ankle, given three times a day for four days, then night and morning for three days, after which the situation is reassessed. When pain is centred at the insertion of the Achilles tendon, Ruta Graveolens 30c given in the same way is usually effective. Rhus Tox. is also commonly indicated when the symptoms of backache caused by injury are aggravated on first movement, and relieved by subsequent movement. In such cases manipulative treatment may also be required. To relieve pain from major operations such as appendicectomy, a combined remedy is often effective. Staphysagria covers pain in a cut wound. Bellis Perennis covers injury to soft tissue. A combined dose of the 200c potency is given before operation, and repeated, say, three times daily post-operatively. When there is pain in a cut wound, Staphysagria 200c is usually successful.

Pain in scars caused by injury, including operation, can often be dealt with by homoeopathic remedies chosen on their individual indications. There is, however, one remedy which can often be successful – Thiosinaminum, prepared from oil of mustard seed, and given in the 200c potency. A woman of forty had suffered from mastitis for many years, despite extensive conventional treatment. I treated her with Sepia 30c, which was individually indicated. Shortly after this a carbuncle formed on the outer side of the left breast, which discharged leaving a large scar and painful adhesions. Thiosinaminum 200c was given and successfully dealt with the pain of the adhesions. Unknown to me, this patient had had an appendicectomy at the age of twenty, and since then had suffered considerable pain in the right iliac fossa if she rose quickly from a seat. After taking the Thiosinaminum she was surprised to find that this recurrent pain also disappeared and never returned.

Chapter 2

The Homoeopathic Approach

Several years ago a child was admitted to Barton Ward suffering from diphtheria, which was confirmed by a throat swab. The child was transferred to a fever hospital next day after having been given Merc. Cyan. 200c. The fever hospital sent the child home as their throat swab was negative. We were informed that we had made a wrong diagnosis. Mentioning this to Dr Borland, he told me that this was not an unusual happening. On one occasion the Superintendent of the fever hospital actually came round at Dr Borland's invitation to see the laboratory evidence. All he said was that 'there must have been a mistake somewhere'.

It is hard to believe the ignorance about homoeopathy in the medical profession and still more in those responsible for the education of medical students. In an address to the British Medical Association Dr Charles Wheeler said: 'To say that the vast body of medical opinion for a hundred years has rejected homoeopathy is true, but to imply that it has rejected it after trial and investigation is a gross fallacy. Each successive decade has handed its prejudice and ignorance on to the next, and the simple tests which would have settled the matter once and for all have never been made, save by the few, who in consequence have maintained the heresy.'

Minute or infinitesimal doses of drugs which are commonly prescribed in homoeopathic practice constitute the most formidable mental obstacle for doctors, so that they do not give homoeopathy a second thought. Students are taught exclusively the use of drugs for their direct chemical or physical effects, and for these purposes adequate doses are obviously necessary. Not being given the facts about homoeopathy, the vast majority of doctors, in the UK at any rate, imagine that homoeopathy consists of such treatment as giving a millionth of a grain of aspirin instead of five grains to relieve a headache, or an infinitesimal dose of penicillin to cure pneumonia, which would of course be absurd. The word homoeopathy means 'like sickness', and as this implies, homoeopathic treatment consists broadly speaking in administering a medicine which is capable in health of evoking symptoms similar to those representing the patient's reaction to illness.

It is difficult for anyone trained in the more orthodox use of drugs to see this as a reality, yet homoeopathy has survived for the greater part of two centuries – despite much opposition – simply because it has given satisfactory results.

Take measles, for example. One child is irritable, intensely thirsty, dislikes interference, especially being moved; another craves affection, is weepy, and is thirstless during the height of fever. Other children may respond in other ways. It is known that Bryonia is capable of evoking in health the kind of reaction of the first child, and Pulsatilla that of the second. The homoeopathic treament of the first child would be Bryonia, and of the second child Pulsatilla. It is not the size of the dose which makes a medicine homoeopathic, but the grounds (of similarity) on which it is selected. Hahnemann and his pupils practised homoeopathy for ten years with material doses of drugs, before using potentized medicines – which erroneously have been taken for weak or inadequate doses of medicine.

This is discussed shortly, but it should be made clear that it is only in respect of medicines chosen in this way that there is any question of giving potentised drugs. All experienced doctors and nurses know how different patients react in different ways to any acute infectious disease. Reactions of the Bryonia and Pulsatilla kind are fairly common, whether it is measles or primary pneumonia or typhoid fever. Such symptom complexes are not directly caused by the pathological process, and it is reasonable to regard them as in some way representing the patient's attempt to get well. It is well known that when resistance is low – both in the very young and the very old, in the under-twos and the over-eighties – the effects of antibiotic treatment are not so good as in the in-between age groups. It is, we believe, this factor which can be influenced by homoeopathic treatment.

Some years ago Dr Priestman and I had the opportunity to treat some hundreds of cases of pneumonia in the Children's Ward. We had between forty and fifty admissions each year of primary pneumonia. A few had had penicillin before they were admitted, and in some we used penicillin, but over 90 per cent were treated solely by homoeopathy. In moribund cases penicillin was given as well as homoeopathy, the first to damp down infection and the second in an attempt to raise resistance. Oxygen was of course administered on the usual clinical indications. It was suggested that it might be worth while to treat half the patients with homoeopathy and the other half with penicillin. Obviously, such an experiment would be of little value unless many more cases were studied in this way, and cases would have to be selected on grounds of age and severity, etc. In any case, we felt certain that one child could be lost because of lack of penicillin and another might die from lack of homoeopathy. Even if we could prove the value of homoeopathy, such an outcome would have been at too great a cost.

In the early part of this century, Dr Robertson Day studied the statistics of pneumonias treated at the London Homoeopathic Hospital and in other London hospitals. He claimed that the mortality rate was 50 per cent lower in the Homoeopathic Hospital, but, and this is the interesting point, he claimed that the death rate in children was still lower. The advantage of antibiotic treatment is that they do not require special training to adminster, but the disadvantage is that their value depends on the nature of the infectious micro-organism. Homoeopathy can be applied immediately, and there are no problems of this kind as a general rule. Also there are no side effects. In other words, our attitude was that if it were possible to cure without danger of side effects, that would be the treatment of choice. In very severe cases, or cases not responding, or in which the homoeopathic medicine was not easy to find, both were given.

Every now and then some leading member of the medical profession seems to feel it his bounden duty to make derogatory remarks about homoeopathy. Although these self-appointed judges do not have much knowledge of homoeopathy, and certainly have never tested it out properly, their influence is such that many honest members of the profession are still further dissuaded from looking into the subject.

A few years ago a medical professor whose name I forget suggested that those who practise homoeopathy give it to patients who have nothing seriously wrong, but when a patient is seriously ill the homoeopaths know full well that 'proper' treatment must be given. No claim has ever been made that homoeopathy is capable of curing everything. Hahnemann himself taught that it would be absurd not to use treatment other than homoeopathy when conditions warranted it, including surgery, which he advocated even in its crude state at that time – for example, in the removal of a stone in the bladder.

Not infrequently doctors argue about homoeopathy on such false assumptions that one has to explain to them what they are really discussing, and even then misunderstanding is usually so deeply ingrained that you end up hearing something about faith and suggestion, natural cure and the personality of the doctor!

Towards the end of the eighteenth century, prescriptions of up to two dozen ingredients were sometimes prescribed, in the hope, as someone put it, that at least one would hit the mark. There was a flourishing trade in unicorn's horns, and it is no wonder that Hahnemann was fiercely attacked by the Chemists' Guilds. The insane were beaten to drive off evil spirits, and many patients were purged or bled to death.

Hahnemann's first experiment was with cinchona bark – crude quinine – which was one of the few specifics available. Malaria was prevalent in Germany at that time. After taking therapeutic doses of cinchona bark Hahnemann developed symptoms resembling malaria. He continued to experiment on his family and friends with cinchona bark and several other drugs to find their effects in health. Then, when a patient presented himself whose symptom complex resembled such known drug effects, Hahnemann tried out the appropriate drug therapeutically and noted the results. It has been said that Hahnemann might well have happened to develop malaria after taking the cinchona bark, and it has even been said that he built a system of therapeutics on a single misleading experiment. But Hahnemann was an experienced investigator and was the last man to be deceived in that way. It was only after six years of such experiments that he published an essay on a new way of discovering the curative power of drugs.

The only reference I had to homoeopathy as an undergraduate was by Dr Clarke, Professor of Materia Medica and Therapeutics at the University of Edinburgh. He gave Hahnemann credit for being the first to put pharmacology on an experimental basis, but added that when it came to the question of doses the whole thing became ridiculous. Professor Clarke said that in a 200th potency of Natrum Sulph. there would be a single molecule of the drug in a volume of diluent equal to the size of the known universe, and the chances of your patient getting that molecule in her bottle was correspondingly small! That must have been the end of homoeopathy for thousands of students who passed through his otherwise capable hands. It probably would have been for me also if it were not for the fact that I was paired with a science student in the class of practical physiology, who told me of alleged cures of friends of his by homoeopathic treatment when orthodox treatment had failed. He was a keen Rugby footballer and he found that Arnica Montana took out most of the aches and pains after the first game of the season. (It is interesting to note that the German and Russian armed forces used Arnica to help deal with shock in battle casualties in World War Two.) I did some reading about homoeopathy, and the idea of giving medicines with the object of stimulating the patient to get well appealed to me so strongly that I decided to find out whether it worked or not. Dr Henderson Patrick, then Senior Physician of the Glasgow Homoeopathic Hospital, to whom I applied for guidance, said, 'Wait till you have qualified and then we will teach you.'

I could not wait, however, and experimented on my family and friends as occasion arose, but my first efforts were not very successful. There was only one apparently striking success. A man of just over 70 was severely ill with influenza. It was just after I had qualified. He had delusions of being scattered about in the bed. His daughter told me that it was unlikely anything more could be done – this was, as she put it, 'the break-up', which, by a coincidence, had also preceded the death of two other members of the family. Baptisia has that kind of delirium, and after a few doses of the 200th potency he made a rapid recovery and lived for another seven years.

The question of potentised drugs has led to much confusion. There was nothing in Hahnemann's early experiments to indicate the size of the dose. He noted, especially in chronic disease, that there was sometimes a temporary worsening of the patient's condition. He decided to try to find the optimal dose of each drug, enough to work satisfactorily but without what he regarded as side actions. He diluted his medicines by succussion and found to his surprise that similar medicines worked even better when prepared in this way, and thus the term 'potentised medicines' arose.

It is only very recently that some light has been shed on the power developed in these medicines. It is a fact known to all experienced homoeopaths that highly potentised medicines act more powerfully than crude drugs or even low potencies, in other words, medicines which have not been diluted and succussed to the same extent.

In the early part of this century there was a difference of opinion between homoeopaths who used low potencies and those who believed in high ones. Dr Wheeler compared the results in treatment of some hundred cases of pneumonia and found that the mortality rate was the same, but that patients treated on the high potencies recovered much more quickly. Recent work on 'anomalous' and 'polymerised' water gives support to the view that the effects of potentised medicines may well result from a change in the molecular structure of the solvent. Water molecules form long chains. The length and type of these chains seem to depend on the physical state of the water, the chemical characteristics of which may be determined accordingly. It is also probable that shaking, or succussion, alters these bonds.

Significant was the work done by the late Dr G. P. Barnard, research physicist, and that of Dr J. H. Stephenson in New York. Their joint paper on the subject, completed in 1965, said in part in its summary: 'Recent application of quantum chemistry theory to biological systems indicates that these succussed high dilutions may act via the physico-dynamic structure of their solvent phase, rather than the chemical properties of their dissolved solutes. The solvent molecules may arrange themselves into stereospecific, isotactic polymers with the ability of self-replication in the absence of the initial exciting solute. Certain physical qualities of these succussed high dilutions appear to verify this conclusion.'

Medicines potentised to the stage referred to by Professor Clarke act powerfully not only on man but also on animals. Pulsatilla 200c has a reputation among farmers for treatment of retained placenta in cattle.

In order to find out more about homoeopathy I obtained an appointment as house surgeon, and later as house physician and eventually as registrar, at the Royal London Homoeopathic Hospital before the war.

It was soon apparent that my early failures were due to my scanty knowledge of the materia medica and virtually no knowledge of homoeopathic case-taking and prescribing. While on the surgical side, I tried out homoeopathy in postoperative cases, especially to try to relieve pain due to flatulence. With expert guidance then freely available, I found that patients who were painfully distended, and who obtained relief from eructations, responded well to Carbo Veg. 200c. Those who got relief from passing flatus usually responded to Lycopodium, and a number of remedies, especially Raphanus 200c were, according to indications, effective in most cases where the wind could not be dispelled in these ways. I used to wait in the evenings after operations, and if I failed to get results I gave morphia or in other ways relieved the patient's distress. One of the more striking effects of homoeopathy was the rapid relief of pain in a patient waiting for operation for a protruding lumbar disc, when large doses of Omnopon had failed, by giving Coffea 10M. In a case of pleurisy not relieved even by morphia, Bryonia 200c gave rapid relief. I gave Arnica to a woman who was complaining bitterly of aching pains caused by a fractured neck of femur. It had no effect. As she was weepy, craving sympathy and I could not think of anything else, I prescribed Pulsatilla 200c. Shortly after she called me as I was passing her bed and said, 'Doctor, that second medicine went straight to the spot.'

Gradually I became convinced of the therapeutic power of homoeo-pathy. When I was acting as house surgeon the children undergoing tonsillectomy were given Arnica before operation and Rhus Tox. 30c afterwards. I had insufficient hospital experience to compare the results with orthodox treatments, but it was obvious that nurses and sisters coming from other hospitals were very impressed with the results in the way of lack of pain postoperatively. As this is the most common operation in children, it provided a basis of comparison. None of the children were denied pain killers.

When acting as Dr Tyler's clinical assistant I saw many interesting cases treated by homoeopathy. For example, a young woman who had been sent home after investigation for a cerebral tumour which proved to be inoperable. She had a plentiful supply of morphia, which had little or no effect. As her health had been undermined by a severe attack of diphtheria, Dr Tyler prescribed Diphtherinum 200c and there was a remarkable easing of pain. The medicine was repeated when pains became severe again with further relief. She lived for several months without much pain. When tackled about the effects of suggestion being mistaken for homoeopathic treatment Dr Tyler used to say, 'Well, if it is, it is a very useful way to apply suggestion.'

There is no recent statistical evidence of the effects of homoeopathic treatment such as there was last century in epidemics of cholera. In an epidemic in London in 1854, the evidence in favour of homoeopathic treatment was overwhelming, as judged by orthodox authorities, but this was not included in a report of the epidemic. When the Member of Parliament responsible was asked about the omission, he said that if he had included it it might have encouraged quackery. The most recent large-scale statistical evidence of the effects of homoeopathic treatment is as far back as the pandemic of influenza following World War I. Homoeopathic doctors in America claimed that their rate of mortality in 17,000 cases of all ages in the second wave of the disease was 0.3 per cent, against an overall mortality of about 20 per cent.

These statistics may be wrong, but any claim to superiority of homoeopathic treatment in the past is put down to the bad effects of orthodox treatment at whatever time the statistics were produced. Although over 10 per cent of medical beds in hospitals are at present occupied by patients suffering from iatrogenic disease, this is still apparently no argument to try out homoeopathy.

Not everyone has the opportunities that I have had in seeing a team of expert homoeopathic physicians at work. If somehow we could overcome the virtual brainwashing of medical students, we should be prepared to make it much easier for inquirers to try out homoeopathy. Unlike testing a new antibiotic or analgesic in one's practice, some preparation and study is necessary before homoeopathy can be properly evaluated clinically.

Could we not concentrate on near specifics such as Arnica for surgical shock, Chamomilla for teething difficulties, Ignatia for recent grief and so on? We could include remedies for animals, such as Graphites for hard pad in dogs for those who have an opportunity to try out homoeopathy in that way. As a medical registrar, one of my duties was to help in teaching the medical officers homoeopathy. It was soon apparent to me that the best way was to ensure that any apparently striking results were seen by the doctors. Then and then only would they take up the study seriously.

Chapter 3

Observations on the Study of Homoeopathy

Newcomers to homoeopathy are confronted with a new and very different materia medica. In homoeopathic practice medicines are given with the object of stimulating the patients' natural curative powers, as opposed to the use of drugs for their chemical or physical effects on man or micro-organisms.

The homoeopathic materia medica and case-taking, which differs from ordinary case-taking in that indications for therapy of the individual patients are considered as well as symptoms of diagnostic importance, should be studied together with homoeopathic prescribing because they are complementary. Acceptance of homoeopathy does not mean rejection of other forms of treatment; it simply means adding another therapeutic skill to those taught in the medical schools.

MATERIA MEDICA

Dr J. H. Clarke, in his introduction to *The Prescriber*, suggested that the best way to commence study of homoeopathy was to take a few commonly used medicines and try to obtain a thorough understanding of them. He recommended the following list in the order of what he considered to be their importance:

1) Sulphur
2) Lycopodium
3) Calcarea Carbonica
4) Arsenicum Album
5) Thuja
6) Nux Vomica
7) Pulsatilla
8) Silica
9) Hepar Sulphuris
10) China
11) Belladonna
12) Bryonia

He went on to say that an accurate knowledge of these remedies would enable the practitioner to deal successfully with the majority of cases he meets, and it would do more than that – it would provide a solid basis on which to build up a knowledge of the rest of the materia medica.

The homoeopathic materia medica comprises the results of drug provings and their therapeutic effects. The argument that a drug was only homoeopathic if it were capable of producing in health symptoms similar to those cured by it is a thing of the past. Clarke and Hering have both emphasized the fact that just as many accurate indications for prescribing – if not more – have been obtained through careful study of curative effects. For example, the craving for sympathy which is so strongly a pointer to Pulsatilla was a clinical finding.

Aurum Metallicum has a splendid curative record in the treatment of undescended testicle, providing it is not ectopic, yet Aurum obviously could not produce the condition.

The extent of the homoeopathic materia medica, together with the fact that every human being is different from all others, means that every thoroughly experienced homoeopath gains a unique knowledge of it. Much invaluable information has been lost through failure to make careful records. Clarke emphasizes this in the introduction to his *Dictionary of Materia Medica* under the heading: 'Authorities', which I quote:

'In addition to the works of Allen and Hering and the *Cyclopaedia of Drug Pathogenesy*, Dr Curie's edition of Jahr's *Materia Medica*, the materia medicas of Lippe and Guernsey, Cowperthwaite's well-known textbook, and many others have been consulted. But the acount of many of the remedies in the *Dictionary* has been compiled from sources inaccessible to the general reader, being scattered up and down the periodical literature of homoeopathy and throughout the writings of original workers, among whom I may name Dr Compton Burnett and Dr Robert T. Cooper as pre-eminent, each in a line of his own. Throughout the *Dictionary* will be found accredited to these authorities many guiding symptoms of their observation, some already recorded in their published works, very many communicated to me in private conversations, and verified by myself in practice. And I am no less indebted to Dr Thomas Skinner for generous help in materia medica studies. Years ago when I was making a special investigation into the action of the high attenuations, Dr Skinner gave me the greatest possible assistance. We went over a large part of the materia medica together, and the notes I then made have been of great service in compiling this work, especially the introductory sections.'

Dr Skinner was one of the outstanding homoeopaths of his time. Dr Tyler, who used all potencies, told me that when Dr Skinner died it was virtually impossible to do anything for the patients attending his outpatient clinics. She, rightly or wrongly, put this down to the extensive use of very high potencies. There is no doubt that high potencies are very powerful, but she believed that they should be used with caution, despite their potentially dramatic effects.

The question of potency is a complex problem, and one which has perplexed the homoeopathic physician for generations. Dr Sankaran has written an excellent review on this subject and I would strongly recommend his pamphlet: 'The Potency Problem'. He has also written a number of booklets on various aspects of homoeopathy, all of which are very well worth reading.

In studying a homoeopathic remedy it is probably best to read it up first in such books as Tyler's *Drug Pictures* and Kent's *Lectures on Materia Medica*, Nash's *Leaders*, Allen's *Keynotes* – older editions – and Guernsey's *Keynotes of the Materia Medica* – books which give drug pictures and descriptions of constitutional types; before going on to Clarke's *Dictionary of Materia Medica* and the larger works of Hering and Allen.

Hahnemann's *Materia Medica Pura* is well worth consulting also, should the remedy be included in it. Such extensive reading is not as formidable as might be thought as there is much repetition of characteristics of the remedy, which helps to imprint them on the memory – and different features may be stressed in different materia medicas, some of which might otherwise be missed. For example, Guernsey emphasizes the extreme sensitivity to touch of boils and abscesses, requiring Hepar Sulph. – and what a valuable pointer this has been. Sometimes there may be other definite indications, and Hepar Sulph. has never failed me when this symptom was present.

After reading through a remedy it is as well to make one's own summary, which very soon gets coloured from personal experience. You will often find that Boericke's *Materia Medica* gives a fairly similar summary. It is a remarkable book of reference which fills a unique place in homoeopathic practice. Boger's *Synoptic Key* is a similar work – not nearly so complete.

Besides materia medica books, there is a wealth of information to be found in homoeopathic journals such as *The British Homoeopathic Journal* and *Homoeopathy*, old and new – and of the old numbers of the latter, those edited by Dr Tyler are of outstanding interest and practical value. The American magazine, *The Homeopathic Recorder*, now extinct, is also a mine of useful information.

A word about constitutional types so prominently featured in Kent's *Lectures on Materia Medica* and some of the other materia medicas. Hahnemann noted that when Pulsatilla was indicated on what he called

15

corporeal symptoms, the remedy seemed to act specially well on a certain constitutional type of patient. He noted the same in respect of Nux Vomica. Hahnemann's followers noted similar relationships between a few of the homoeopathic remedies and human types of personality, including Arsenicum, Phosphorus, Natrum Mur., Lycopodium, Sepia and Silica.

You may note that with the exception of Sepia, these were all included in Clarke's list. This is because these remedies are among the most commonly used in everyday practice. Also, in the teaching of materia medica it is useful to have some sort of easily remembered features of the remedy being described. While the knowledge of the types is of inestimable value, this aspect of homoeopathy may easily be misleading, especially if the implications of Kent's descriptions are not regarded precisely as Hahnemann stated. The important point is that the remedy should be otherwise indicated. The notion that patients should be 'typed' and then given the appropriate medicine is correct only if the patient can really be typed, and if the remedy covers the patient's complaints. Many patients cannot fit into the very few types described. Perfectly healthy athletes could sometimes be fitted accurately into one of these 'types', yet would need no treatment.

It is convenient to deal with case-taking in acute and chronic illness separately, although there is no sharp dividing line.

CASE-TAKING IN ACUTE ILLNESS

These comprise mainly infections, injuries and the acute manifestations of allergic diseases. It should be noted that the word 'symptom' in homoeopathic literature includes signs. To illustrate the approach to case-taking in acute disease I have often taken a case of primary pneumonia. The symptoms can be divided into two groups – those dependent on an inflamed mass within the chest, and symptoms which cannot be explained by the nature of the pathological process.

This second group is known to all experienced nurses and doctors, but is usually disregarded because these symptoms are of no value in selecting a suitable antibiotic. For example, one patient has become irritable, intensely thirsty, tends to lie on the painful side to keep it still, and has a strong aversion to being moved or interfered with in any way. Another may tend to be weepy, craves sympathy, and is thirstless at the height of the fever.

As this second group of symptoms do not depend directly on the pathology, and as they appear along with the disease and disappear when the patient has recovered, it is difficult to explain them except as in some way reflecting the patient's individual reaction in the attempt to get well. Antibiotics do not have nearly as good effects in the very young and the very old, simply because patients on antibiotics cure themselves, having been helped to fight a weakened opponent. In the very young and old, the natural recuperative powers are minimal, and hence the apparent relative inefficiency of antibiotics.

The homoeopathic remedy is a substance which from its known effects in health is capable of evoking a similar sort of reaction, or is known to have therapeutic actions to that effect. In other words, homoeopathic treatment is selected with the object of giving a boost to the natural defence mechanism which reflects itself in the individual symptom complex.

On these grounds Bryonia is indicated homoeopathically for the first case, and Pulsatilla for the second. If the disease were measles or typhoid fever – and there is much evidence of the efficacy of homoeopathy in both diseases – and the patient reacted in the way calling for Bryonia, that would still be the remedy – and the same applies to Pulsatilla.

Fortunately, there is a tendency for patients suffering from acute illness to react in a limited number of ways, although remedy selection must be accurate. Dr D. M. Borland has written a pamphlet on the treatment of pneumonia, giving the more commonly indicated remedies in his vast experience. Dr Tyler has written some excellent pamphlets on the treatment of colds, coughs, and other acute illnesses, which are very useful for the beginner.

Antibiotic treatment is therefore complementary to the homoeopathic approach and they can be given simultaneously. If there is immediate danger to life I should certainly consider giving both. Otherwise the advantage of homoeopathic treatment is that resistance can be raised against any micro-organism, and there is no danger of side effects.

The golden rule in case-taking with the object of discovering the homoeopathic remedy is to allow the patient to express himself in his or her own way without interruption. He should be allowed to paint his own clinical picture. If the patient is a child, the mother or someone who knows the child very well is best fitted to give the history. If the patient is allowed freedom to speak, it is surprising how often characteristic features of a remedy are presented. Interrupting the patient results in him losing his train of thought, and he often gives the answers he thinks the doctor wants rather than giving the doctor what he really wants – an accurate account of the clinical picture as experienced by the patient.

Diagnosis is, of course, made in the usual way from the history, clinical examination and, as required, special investigations.

The next step is to look for really definite or unusual symptoms, whether given by the patient or by onlookers – or symptoms observed by the physician. Although the range of reactive symptoms is extremely large, it had been found that usually there are relatively very few really definite symptoms. Obviously, one has to take care to be sure they reflect a reaction and are not occasioned by, for example, recent grief, or resentment, which have nothing to do with the present complaint – or a desire for fresh air, if the room is stuffy.

From a few really definite symptoms the remedy can usually be found. A mass of vague and indefinite symptoms is virtually useless from the viewpoint of prescribing. Mental and general symptoms – those where the subject of the sentence is 'I' – are of highest value, if definite.

Observation of the patient is of the greatest importance. I deal with this subject in some detail in chapter 7 ('Paediatric Case-taking') and it does not differ essentially from case-taking in adults, at least in acute illness. For example, the patient's position in bed, whether he is restless, the nature and distribution of perspiration, facial appearance, odours of discharges, sweat, urine, stools, etc. Then it is legitimate to ask questions. There is no perfect plan. Case-taking, like other facets of homoeopathy, develops with greater understanding of the materia medica and clinical experience.

It is useful to have some scheme of questioning – and again it should be emphasized that the questioning should come last, and it must be remembered that 'leading questions get misleading answers'. Inquiry could be made as follows to obtain fuller information on symptoms stressed by the patient:

Mode of Onset
Any obvious precipitating cause such as injury, fright, chill, and whether the illness developed slowly or gradually. For instance, it may be difficult to distinguish between Gelsemium and Baptisia, say, in influenza. There are several differences which may be apparent, although sometimes the decision has to be made on the mode of onset. Gelsemium tends to slowly develop acute illnesses, whereas Baptisia is characterised by a sudden onset.

Thirst
Its nature (if present) or absence. Thirst is normally present in fever and is not therefore of any value unless there is something which is really

definitely unusual about it. For example, thirst for sips of hot drinks is characteristic of Arsenicum; thirst for cold drinks is usual in children and if the child wants warm drinks this is a peculiar symptom. There is a danger of being misled by mothers who only give warm drinks as they feel cold drinks may be harmful and, having nothing else to quench their thirst, the children accept them. Children really wanting warm drinks usually require Arsenicum or Lycopodium, but a remedy should never be prescribed on one symptom, and other symptoms must be present – such as the restlessness and fear, especially around midnight, and fear of death, which very often confirm Arsenicum. Other symptoms may confirm Lycopodium. Thirstlessness during fever has many remedies, which are listed in Kent's *Repertory*, but most often in my experience Gelsemium or Pulsatilla will be found to fit the case in other respects.

Modalities
Times and other circumstances of amelioration or aggravation. Times are most important if definite. Modalities affecting the patient as a whole are of higher value, generally speaking, than modalities of particulars.

Concomitants
Symptoms of other parts of the body not necessarily representing the patient's reaction. Complaints which have come on along with the disease, such as excessive flatulence and abdominal distension in a case of pneumonia, might confirm the choice of Lycopodium if otherwise indicated.

Despite this apparently complex approach, if the principles of case-taking are kept in mind to allow so far as possible a natural 'portrait' of the illness to be painted by the patient, and outstanding symptoms of individual reaction noted, the remedy usually becomes apparent. When there are no definite symptoms representing a reaction, Sulphur is indicated.

Case-taking is similar in acute allergic manifestations and in dealing with the after-effects of injuries. Fortunately, there are some near specifics for the immediate after-effects, such as Arnica for shock. There is some useful information on the subject of injuries in Kent's lecture on Hypericum. This could serve as an introduction to the invaluable contribution homoeopathy can make to the immediate and remote effects of injury. Knowledge of a few 'injury remedies' would enable anyone easily to test out homoeopathy and appreciate the reality of medium and high potencies.

The remedy is most often apparent to the experienced homoeopath after obtaining a good history, and repertorisation is seldom needed. Sometimes it is useful to consider symptoms according to a plan which has been used for generations, placing them under the headings: Location (or Tissues), Sensations, Modalities, and Concomitants. Under the heading of Sensations I place such items as discharges, eruptions, etc. Regarding Concomitants, mentals and generals, mental and physical changes such as irritability, extreme chilliness, etc., which have developed just before or after the illness began, if really definite, are of high value.

CASE-TAKING IN CHRONIC DISEASE

Case-taking in chronic disease is not at all easy to summarise accurately, and very different views are held by experienced homoeopaths. First of all, let us consider Hahnemann's theory of chronic disease. This may be briefly summarised as follows:

After ten years of a very thorough study of case histories, Hahnemann came to the conclusion that there were two diseases analogous to syphilis which at first resembled other acute infections, but which became chronic and could be transmitted to the offspring. These he called sycosis, or figwart disease, which he traced to gonorrhoea, and psora – which in his day manifested itself by an extremely itchy vesicular eruption corresponding to the primary sore in syphilis and the urethral discharge in gonorrhoea. He backed his belief by numerous references to the literature of his time, that suppression of these manifestations – especially psora – led to a much more serious state of affairs. Apart from external adverse influences such as injury and poisoning, he believed that all chronic disease was caused basically by psora, plus or minus one or both of the other 'miasms', as he termed them – the underlying dyscrasia then being lit up by some comparatively trivial inadequacy of diet, chill, emotional stress, etc., and leading to all chronic diseases.

It is interesting to note that one of the many postulates as to the cause of disseminated sclerosis is that some acquired or inherited virus infection of the central nervous system is awakened into activity by such circumstances, and it is noteworthy that there is considerable evidence that this disease is more common in colder climates. Hahnemann then developed new remedies to cope with these chronic infections, in an attempt to cure all that was curable by medicine in chronic disease. His theory has been the subject of controversy for over a century among those who practise homoeopathy.

Dr Tyler and others thought that Hahnemann's psora possibly represented any acute infection which produced a lasting adverse influence on health.

An account of the symptomatology of the miasms can be found in Hempel's translation of Hahnemann's *Chronic Diseases*. Roberts in his book *The Principles and Art of Cure by Homoeopathy* gives a more easily read account. It is perhaps unfortunate that Roberts inserts his own theory, but this does not detract from his delineation of the symptomatology of the miasms. A very comprehensive account of the miasms can be found in J. H. Allen's *Chronic Miasms*. Some knowledge of the miasms is needed to understand homoeopathic materia medica, in which there is frequent reference to them, and it is of practical importance in prescribing.

Hahnemann described his methods of case-taking in the *Organon*, and several attempts to give guidance on this important aspect of homoeopathic practice have been made. Clarke gave his account of case-taking in the preface to *The Prescriber*, and Roberts also gives a useful account of case-taking in *The Principles and Art of Cure by Homoeopathy*.

Each experienced homoeopath tends to develop his own way of case-taking. It is not easy to describe the subject accurately and comprehensively. In case it may be useful to those commencing the study of homoeopathy, I attempt very briefly to outline case-taking in chronic disease.

Present Complaint

The difference is that the patient is allowed to paint his or her own clinical picture in the manner described in respect of acute illness, filled in by observation and very careful questioning so as not to spoil the accurate delineation of the individual features of the illness.

Past History

Bearing in mind the essence of Hahnemann's theory of chronic disease, it is necessary to inquire whether there was any severe acute infection such as measles or influenza from which the patient has not apparently fully recovered, either associated with the onset of the present illness or further back. There is ample evidence that the use of nosodes of acute illness may be invaluable. It is also well worth while to find out if there are any other outstanding episodes in the history, including injury, emotional disturbance, sunstroke, severe reaction to inoculation, drugs or anaesthesia.

Family History
Occasionally we obtain a history of venereal disease, although this is exceptional. I inquire about cancer, tuberculosis and diabetes, as a strong family history of one or more of these suggests consideration of Carcinosin. Occasionally there is a family history of alcoholism, which suggests consideration of Lueticum.

Individual Characteristics and Constitutional Types
Sometimes there is a clear-cut time of commencement of the illness. In such circumstances any mental and general changes developing along with the disease, not always easy to find, may be invaluable, as concomitants and the case can be dealt with in much the same way as acute illness. Often there is an insidious onset, or it may have been long ago and such information is lacking. While taking the history the patient can be observed, and much useful information can be obtained in this way.

Questions may be asked later, with the same precautions to avoid obtaining a false picture. What we want to know is – how does this individual differ in definite ways from a theoretical norm of the same age, sex and social environment? For example, a wrinkled forehead and loss of memory is common in old age, but it would be outside the norm if found in a child. It is worthwhile to find out about likes and dislikes for food, reaction to environment, heat and cold, open air, sea air, thunderstorms, etc., as well as the mental make-up of the patient. Again, we are after really definite symptoms, and if there is any doubt as to whether a symptom is outside the norm it is better to discard it and look for something which is definite. In difficult cases I go over the notes and write out the case history in three columns:
1) Mentals and generals.
2) Present complaint, with all relevant information.
3) Serial history – family history and outstanding events in the history of the patient.

There is nothing new in this but it provides a useful record for reference. Some items might come into more than one column. A rough guide to the strength of a symptom is given by a suitable underlining. Quite often a patient will be seen to belong to one of the recognised constitutional types. I begin to repertorise the symptoms of the present illness. It happens that the remedy for the type covers the present illness as well, that is good grounds for its prescription, but it is not a necessity. Again, the past history may give a very clear pointer, but it is better to attempt to prescribe symptomatically. Only if that fails, or there are no very clear-cut indications, would I give the appropriate nosode or other medicine in that category related to outstanding past events in the history.

REPERTORIES

It is essential to be able to use a repertory. Kent's *Repertory* is generally agreed to be the best, but whatever repertory is used one must be thoroughly familiar with it so that any rubric can be quickly found.

Chapter 4

Constitutional Types

Hahnemann observed that when Pulsatilla was indicated on what he termed 'corporal' symptoms, an especially good effect could be expected when certain mental and emotional changes had taken place since the illness began, and he described the type of patient likely to produce such changes. He also noted that Nux Vomica when so indicated had a particularly beneficial influence on certain types of patient. Other medicines have subsequently been found to act in this way, including Arsenicum Alb., Calc. Carb., and Sepia. That is to say, a number of medicines used in homoeopathic practice have been discovered to act specially well on certain types or groups of human beings, when other indications are also present. These remedies with a facet or facets related in this way to human types are to be found almost exclusively among the polychrests. For this reason, although they are comparatively few, they are of importance out of all proportion to their numbers.

In introducing the materia medica, it is natural that the polychrests, including those linked to constitutional types, receive much attention. A false impression may be engendered that in prescribing for chronic disease the patient must be 'typed', and that the appropriate remedy is the one related to that type. For example, Kent goes much further than Hahnemann in dealing with Pulsatilla. He says, 'The Pulsatilla patient is an interesting one, found in any household where there are plenty of young girls. She is tearful, plethoric, and has little credit for being sick from her appearance: yet she is most nervous, fidgety, changeable, easily led and easily persuaded. While she is mild, gentle and tearful, yet she is remarkably irritable, not in the sense of pugnacity but easily irritated, extremely touchy, always feels slighted or fears she will be slighted; sensible to every social influence, melancholia, sadness, weeping, despair, religious despair. Fanatical, full of notions and whims; imaginative; extremely excitable. She imagines the company of the opposite sex is a dangerous thing to cultivate, that it is dangerous to do certain things well established in human society as good for the human race. These imaginations belong to eating as well as thinking. They imagine that milk is not good to drink, so they will not take it. They imagine that certain articles of diet are not good for the human race. Aversion to marriage is a strong symptom.'

In his lecture on Sulphur Kent says, 'The Sulphur patient is a lean, lank, hungry, dyspeptic fellow with round shoulders, yet many times it is given to fat rotund well-fed people.' He goes on to say 'There is another class of patient in whom we see a Sulphur appearance in the face; dirty, shrivelled, red-faced people. The skin seems to be easily affected by atmosphere. He becomes red in the face from riding in the air both in very cold and in damp weather. He has a delicate thin skin, blushing on the slightest occasion, always red and dirty-looking no matter how much he washes it. If it be a child the mother has to wash the face often, but it always looks as if it had been perfunctorily washed.' Kent then quotes Hering who described the Sulphur patient as the ragged philosopher, and gives another picture of Sulphur types.

Dr Tyler writes: 'It is imperative to get a true realisation of Sepia, one of our most important remedies in chronic diseases. She continues, 'I am told that Dr Gibson Miller, the great prescriber, used to say that if he might have only one drug, he would choose Sepia. And Sepia has made some wonderful cures, when the unit dose has been left to act over several months: goitre, insanity, rheumatoid arthritis, etc.' Now how to spot Sepia . . . 'Sepia has been called the washerwoman's remedy and not without cause. Picture her – the sallow, tired mother of a large family, on 'washing day'. She is perspiring profusely; pouring under the arms. She cannot be shut in, because of the heat and the stuffiness which makes her feel faint – yet the cold wind that rushes in at the open window is almost unbearable. Her back aches fearfully. She wants to press it – to support it (Natrum Mur.). She feels she must sit down, or cross her legs, as her whole inside seems to be dragging down, and coming out of her. She simply must sit down to keep it in (Lilium Tig.).

'The worry of the children is more than she can bear. Her Chamomilla baby wants to be picked up and carried, and wails and screams. The quarrels of the penultimate babies, engaged in scratching each other's eyes out, are more than she can bear. And when her 6-year old starts drumming with a spoon on a tin pot, she can stand it no more. She snatches the tin pot and hurls it away and smacks her small son; which does not improve matters. He howls dismally and she does not care. Oh how she wants to run away and leave it all and have a little peace. Her head aches. The pain is left-sided today; last time it was on the right side, as she remembers dully. She is so jumpy and nervous, she has to hold on to the edge of the wash-tub to prevent herself from screaming. If she could only go away from everybody and everything, and lie down, alone in the dark, and close her eyes! Her husband comes in: she has no smile to greet his. Nothing but dull indifference, and weariness, and suffering. He must leave her alone.

She has her work to do. Ptosis, ptosis everywhere. Her whole body is dragged down, 'inside' and out. Veins – piles – all stagnant and dragging her down. Even her eyelids are too heavy to hold up. If only she could lie down and close them. She knows even ten minutes' sleep would make her a new woman. But there are the soapsuds – the steam – the stuffiness – the terrors of her restless children with their noise and fidgeting. Sleep is not for her. Her little Pulsatilla maid creeps up, 'Can't I help you Mummy?' but she pushes her off. And the little maid creeps away, weeping; and Mummy feels that she is indifferent to her tears. The dinner is cooking, and the smell of cooking makes her feel deadly sick. The children are hungry and her husband waits for his dinner. She is indifferent. Let them wait. She is irritable, indifferent and apathetic. He looks at her sadly. Her dull face has lost its contour – its bloom – its pleasing lines. Browny bands or blotches are on her forehead and saddle-wise across nose and cheekbones. She was a bright and bonny girl when he married her – now she is Sepia.'

It is understandable that such descriptions may tend to mislead those not fully trained in homoeopathic prescribing.

While such 'clinical imagery', as Kent put it, is necessary to introduce the materia medica, he stressed that the only way to grasp the essence of a drug was to read and re-read the provings. It should be remembered too that some of the polychrests have not been found to have links with human types, for example, Rhus Tox. and Bryonia, not to mention hundreds of remedies other than the polychrests.

Not all patients, then, can be fitted into recognised types, and to fit a patient into a type to which he does not belong is obviously a wrong approach. There is also the danger that prescription of the wrong remedy in this category, especially in high potency, may have some effect, because the polychrests have a widespread influence on man. Results may be sufficiently good to encourage the practice of fitting patients into types as a preliminary to constitutional prescribing.

The fact that anyone can be fitted into a type, even accurately, does not mean that the remedy for that type is required at any given time. If you were to take a sufficient number of perfectly healthy athletes, there would be representatives of every recognised type, and many who could not be fitted into any known type.

Then consider what might happen if a person who was previously in excellent health, whether belonging to a recognised type or not, became ill. Take acute conditions, for instance primary pneumonia. Symptoms common to the disease are of lowest value in homoeopathic prescribing. It is the individual symptoms, those reflecting the patient's reaction to the illness which are of almost exclusive importance in selecting the remedy, such as the mode of onset, mental and physical changes which have occurred since pneumonia began, and modalities. One patient is irritable, wants long drinks and dislikes to be disturbed or moved. He may lie on the affected side to try and keep still, as movement aggravates the pain. Another is frightened and restless, worse after midnight and wants sips of warm fluids. Bryonia is capable of evoking in health a symptom complex similar to those exhibited by the first patient and Arsenicum Alb. the second. Homoeopathic treatment would consist in giving the first patient Bryonia and the second Arsenicum Alb. To put it in another way, having observed the pattern of response as reflected in the individual symptoms which cannot be explained on a pathological basis, a suitable individual stimulus is administered which is known to be capable of producing that kind of reaction.

This approach is applicable to other acute conditions, although certain acute diseases call for a virtually specific remedy, such as Arnica for surgical shock and Ignatia for acute grief. A limited number of remedies cover the vast majority of patients suffering from some acute illness, for instance, Drosera, Coccus Cacti and Kali Carb. in the treatment of whooping cough, presumably because there is tendency to react in a limited number of ways to a specific stimulus. It does not matter what type, known or unknown, the patient may have been before the onset of the acute illness; it is the recently-developed symptoms on which the prescription is based. Generally speaking it is better to avoid a constitutional medicine previously related to the patient, except some-times during convalescence, or in the sub-acute stage, and only if indicated on symptoms present.

Then consider a previously healthy person who develops a chronic illness. Although Dr Tyler's Sepia patient was a fictitious one intended to describe the Sepia type, or the group of patients who have by experience been found to respond well to Sepia, it serves well to illustrate the value of a knowledge of remedy-sensitive types. Dr Tyler did not say whether the patient could have been classified as previously belonging to one of the known types or not. This in fact does not matter. The position that was the totality of symptoms present were covered by Sepia and it so happened that the patient could be recognised as belonging to a group of individuals who respond especially well to Sepia. If the patient's symptoms were covered by Sepia and the patient could not be placed in the Sepia group, Sepia would still be the right remedy.

When starting to practise homoeopathy I was puzzled to find a patient, a young woman, who suffered from chronic sinusitis; her symptoms were completely covered by Sepia, yet she could not be fitted into the descriptions of Sepia which I had at that time mistakenly believed to form an essential ingredient of the indications for Sepia in chronic conditions. Sepia, however, cured the patient. (Hahnemann made no reference to constitutional prescribing in his *Chronic Diseases*.)

Hahnemann's teaching on case-taking was very briefly summarised by Boenninghausen, and this extreme abbreviation was also taught by Hering, who used to put on the blackboard the well-known drawing illustrating the information necessary for a homoeopathic prescription; namely, location of tissues, sensation, modalities and concomitants. This may appear at first sight to be diametrically opposed to Kent's teaching of working from generals to particulars, but if one remembers that concomitants mean mentals and generals, with special value placed on recent changes, it will be apparent that the totality of symptoms can be arrived at by either of these approaches. Some cases lend themselves to one approach and some to the other.

Sometimes there are no very clear-cut indications for the remedy in patients previously healthy who have developed chronic disease. In these circumstances, or when apparently well-indicated medicines fail to produce satisfactory results, and the onset is associated with some acute episode, the appropriate nosode or other remedy related to the mode of onset may achieve results. It is not by any means always easy to prescribe in this way. For example, a woman may not have been well since parturition. We are then faced with the decision as to whether the prescription needs to be based on physical trauma, the effects of drugs, including anaesthetics, emotional disturbance, etc. There is, however, no doubt at all that sometimes the results of such an approach may be dramatic. This means that in some way or other the prescription has effectively dealt with recent changes. The type of the patient before the illness, whether belonging to one of the recognised groups or not, seems to be of no practical value in deciding on the prescription.

Some patients seem to be classifiable as belonging to one of the types as far back as one can reasonably ascertain. While all types tend to change in response to acute illness, chronic disease may be met with in such patients without alteration in type, and the whole clinical picture, the recently developed symptom complex included, is covered by the type remedy also.

A woman of 45 complained of migraine of twenty years' duration. She was of the Sepia type so far as I could judge all her life, and the head-aches were also covered by Sepia. She was almost completely free from headaches after treatment by Sepia given at long intervals. A dose of Carcinosin, which is complementary to Sepia, completed the cure.

On the other hand there is evidence that most, if not all, people tend to change their constitutional type. Apart from hereditary influences, and if you like, karmic and extra-terrestrial influences, the developing embryo is subjected to many potential hazards, including injury, infection, drugs and radiation. At birth there is also injury, perhaps drugs, including anaesthetics, and possibly emotional disturbance, when one comes to think of the very close link between mother and infant. There is the likelihood of constitutional changes from one or more of these influences.

Constitutional changes following various infections are discussed by Kent in his lecture on Baryta Carb. He says, 'When a child has almost any disease – measles, scarlet fever, mumps, or even a bad cold, or a malarial attack, the development ceases and dwarfishness results, a state in which he was not born but a state he has acquired.' Tyler's Sepia patient represents a not uncommon way in which constitution may change in response to the stress of numerous pregnancies and the bringing up of young children. Another illustration of constitutional change is the tendency for certain remedies to be more often required at certain phases of life, in childhood, at puberty, at the menopause and in old age. Dr Borland wrote a booklet on *Children's Types*, although he was fully conversant with the treatment of patients of all ages.

To summarise. Certain remedies employed in homoeopathic practice appear to produce especially good results when given to related constitu-tional types of patients. Many patients cannot be so classified.

These remedies are very few in number, but as they are to be found almost exclusively among the polychrests they are of great practical importance.

In introducing the materia medica, clinical imagery, including descrip-tions of such types, plays an important part and this is liable to lead to a misunderstanding. There is a danger that the inexperienced may attempt to fit patients into types as a preliminary to constitutional prescribing.

If the totality of symptoms are covered, the correct prescription can almost always be found. If it should happen that the patient can be classified as belonging to a known group or type at the time of the prescription, this could be an additional indication, but it is not a necessity.

Constitution is liable to change from conception onwards, and it does not matter what type (known or unknown) the patient may have been prior to the onset of the illness under consideration.

Finally, a quotation from Dr Douglas Ross: 'The ever-present danger is that one narrows down the field of search to the few polychrests whose characteristics are best known. To define a patient as belonging to a certain remedy-sensitive group is not to say he needs that remedy at the moment. The totality of symptoms, indeed the departure from his usual method of reacting to environment must determine the choice.'

Chapter 5

The Significance of Past History

Constitutional Treatment

Constitutional homoeopathic treatment consists mainly of prescribing on the psychosomatic make-up of the patient and on the past history. The patient is viewed against a background of a theoretical average person of the same age, sex and social environment, and the salient mental and physical characteristics are noted and matched by a remedy having a similar drug picture. One or more, usually a number of remedies carefully chosen in this way, can frequently restore health when there are no insuperable pathological barriers. Quite often the psychosomatically selected remedy can cover outstanding episodes in the past, for example Natrum Mur. when the patient has had concussion. However, sometimes it seems that it is necessary directly to antidote some past event which greatly disturbed the patient's health. The patient's past history and the family history are similarly viewed against the background of a theoretical average family and personal history, and outstanding features or events are noted. Then, if psychosomatic prescribing fails to produce satisfactory results, the past history may lead to an appropriate remedy for that individual. Alternatively, it may be advisable to prescribe on the family or individual history when there are no clear symptomatic indications for any one remedy right from the beginning.

Observations on the Homoeopathic Materia Medica

Failure to achieve results is usually put down to incorrect prescribing, very often quite rightly, but it should be appreciated that the homoeopathic materia medica is incomplete. There are no records of any unsuccessful proving in over a century and a half, which suggests that all, or nearly all, substances on earth are capable of affecting man in the potentised, if not in the crude state; which means that there are several thousand potential homoeopathic remedies as yet untouched. Even if the almost insuperable difficulties of proving and clinically testing were overcome, the addition of so many new medicines would tend to offset

31

any gains by making the already unwieldy and complex materia medica so large that it would be virtually impossible for anyone to become familiar with it. The difficulties of remedy selection would be even greater than they are at present. The immense field covered by the existing materia medica is surprising, however the selection was made.

The only way that appreciable progress can be made through provings is to be able to predetermine the potential value of the substance to be proved. However difficult the problem, much more thought must be given to it. Most recent provings have been almost entirely wasted, because there is little incentive to carry out an intensive clinical trial of a remedy which might in the end turn out to be of very little value, although the provings themselves have been carried out scientifically and with the utmost care. Clinical testing is necessary to provide the more important part of the remedy picture.

In the meantime, the best possible use should be made of the valuable materia medica available, and careful attention to past history is the one way by which this can be achieved. Also, in view of the limitations of the proved and tested materia medica, there should be no hesitation in pre-scribing unproved remedies, such as the nosodes of acute disease, as occasion demands.

This is not intended to imply that the vast resources of the homoeopathic materia medica of thoroughly tested remedies should be in any way neglected, or that the exacting discipline of remedy selection on a symptomatic basis can be escaped. The object of this chapter is rather to draw attention to the value sometimes obtainable from the patient's past history, and to justify the administration of unproved potentised medicines in certain specified circumstances.

Not Well Since. . .

Chronic ill-health may follow a severe acute or chronic infection, injury, emotional upset or, occasionally, after adverse effects of drugs. Apart from demonstrable pathological sequelae, the patient's vitality – the general level of health – may be lowered. It is often possible by constitutional prescribing to raise the patient's vitality to the extent that functional disorders and diseases with reversible pathological changes may be cured. It is sometimes also possible to help in this way, to some extent, even in incurable conditions.

Acute Infection

When a patient is slow in recovering from any acute infection, certain remedies, such as Sulphur, Psorinum and Carbo Veg., suggest themselves, although the prescription must be selected individually. In these circumstances, or when prolonged ill-health follows, the nosodes of acute infection may be invaluable. Kent and others have rightly condemned the indiscriminate use of nosodes. The place of nosodes in acute infections is fairly clear. They should be considered (a) in the absence of satisfactory indications for a proved remedy, and (b) when remedies apparently well chosen on a symptomatic basis fail to achieve adequate results.

Swan of America was the first to use nosodes extensively, and among his followers may be included Allen, Compton Burnett and Tyler.

Dr Tyler, writing on Morbillinum, said, 'Swan, pioneer in the use of disease products for the cure of like disease, received the inspiration and prepared, among many such substances, potentised measles, with which he did some astonishing work. And now, after all these years of dullness and neglect, we are receiving fresh impetus and are already getting astonishing results. For years we have been making play with Variolinum, Tuberculinum, Lueticum, Medorrhinum, Influenzinum; Morbillinum and several others have till now not entered into the picture, and Morbillinum threatens to become the most important of the lot. Everybody has had measles, and not everybody has managed to 'annihilate the disease' so that nothing latent and threatening has remained. In future we shall do well to take notice when told of an old acute sickness: 'Never, or very tardily, recovered from . . ., never well since diphtheria – scarlet fever – vaccination.' 'Tonsillitis followed by chorea, even rheumatism; heart damaged in childhood by rheumatic fever'. These last put in a strong plea for that mighty remedy Streptococcin.

Having worked with Dr Tyler for some years, I was able to observe her results at first hand, and they were certainly often remarkable. My impression is that her success was to some considerable extent due to careful constititutional prescribing before giving the nosode. Many of the patients had received her expert treatment for years beforehand, but she did prescribe the appropriate nosode at the beginning if there were no obvious indications for a proved remedy, and her results then also were usually very good.

Apart from the probable advantage of careful constitutional prescribing prior to giving the appropriate nosode, there is another reason why these nosodes should be given only after due consideration. That is – they may work like a charm, or not at all. The same applies to administration of a potency of any which has adversely affected a patient.

Tyler published a number of her cases in *Homoeopathy*. Here is one under the title 'Rheumatism – Scarlatina'. I have abbreviated the notes. 'November 1939. Patient sent by her doctor with request for 'massage for her legs and feet for rheumatism'. She had had rheumatic pains for two years. Symptoms were indefinite as regards choice of remedy, but she had had scarlet fever as a child and it had left her with a 'bad ear'. Rx Scarlatinum 200c, three doses 6 hourly (Tyler's favourite prescription of the nosodes), no massage.' In December 1939 there is a note: 'Walking better. Pain gone from legs. Better in herself.' Scarlatinum was repeated in February 1940 and again in October 1940, when Tyler wrote, 'The nosode was repeated as before. This was her second repeat in eleven months in which she has been practically well of two years' rheumatism. She has never needed or been given massage.'

I had a case of this sort a few years ago, when no remedy seemed clearly indicated from the start. A university student had been unable to concentrate and suffered from attacks of vertigo when walking. He described this as feeling 'as if he had put one foot in a small boat'. This began after an attack of measles two years previously. The cause of the vertigo was obscure, he had been checked over at the ENT department of a teaching school without a definite diagnosis having been made. Morbillinum 200c, one dose, was followed by a short aggravation, then complete cure.

Apart from the nosodes of acute childish and other illnesses, it is worth while to note any tendency to streptococcal, staphylococcal or any bacterial or virus infection.

Tyler mentioned Streptococcin in relation to a rheumatic fever history, meaning that such a history would suggest Streptococcin, should there be the indications for a nosode, as a constitutional remedy. Staphylococcal infection is common too, and Staphylococcin may be a useful remedy. A Down's child of eight years suffered from furunculosis of her back and perineum, which was sluggish in responding to treatment. Staphylococcin 30c was followed by a rapid clearing of the condition. Several months later there was a recurrence and again Staphylococcin 30c cleared it up, and it is still clear after some months.

A lad of 15 years of age had suffered from eczema practically all his life, accompanied by secondary infection on many occasions. It was widespread, and he had been in hospital almost half his life, partly because of the severity of his condition and partly because his home conditions were far from good. He responded slowly and unsatisfactorily to homoeopathic treatment, till it was noted that he was always worse at night. A nightly aggravation is covered by about two hundred remedies, but when this remains an outstanding feature after apparently well-indicated remedies have been given, Lueticum is nearly always required. He was given Leuticum 30c, and this was followed by great improvement. Then a month later he developed widespread furunculosis. Staphylococcin 30c was given and there was a dramatic improvement. Staphylococcin had to be repeated six months later, and he has been practically free from eczema and furunculosis for a year. It is, of course, impossible to assess the part played by Staphylococcin in this case, as Lueticum is associated with 'successions of abscesses', a point also to remember in utilising the past history for prescribing. I mention this case as it illustrates the kind of case in which Staphylococcin seems to be indicated; that is to say, when there have been recurrent staphylococcal lesions over a long period of time and when staphylococcal lesions are widespread. At least it is worth a trial in these circumstances when all else fails. It would take a careful analysis of many cases to establish a 'clinical proving' of Staphylococcin, which I believe would be of value in respect of many of the nosodes of acute infection.

A clinical proving should be based on a large number of cases, say at least fifty. Before publishing the first paper on Carcinosin we had detailed notes of over two hundred patients. Some years ago I made a brief study of Streptococcin from about thirty cases. The most definite symptom which emerged was 'weepy, consolation aggravates', and this has been of value in confirming several subsequent prescriptions. Another symptom which emerged, although not quite so definitely, was 'better in the open air'. Streptococcin also has certain rheumatic symptoms indistinguishable from those of Rhus Tox. and other remedies, which one might expect from its pathological relationship to Pyrogen: 'Worse in wet weather, worse on beginning to move, better for subsequent movement'. A woman of 50 had fallen on her knees and had pain which had persisted for some months, although there was no evidence of a fracture or osteoarthritis. She had these symptoms and Rhus Tox. helped a little. Arnica and Ruta had no obvious effect. Many years previously she had suffered from quinsy and rheumatic fever. Streptococcin 30c, three doses, 2 hourly, was followed by a dramatic and lasting freedom from pain, although she was not completely cured.

Along with these nosodes is a group of remedies with a pathological relationship to certain illnesses, including Thuja, Drosera and Lathyrus Sativa in respect of vaccination, whooping cough and poliomyelitis. Thuja is well known for its importance in dealing with the after-effects of vaccination, immediate or remote, and it can be prescribed much in the same way as a nosode. That is to say, when there are no clear indications for another remedy, or when apparently indicated remedies do not act satisfactorily, even when symptomatic indications are absent. Failure to take after a first vaccination, and even very large vaccination scars, should also lead to consideration of Thuja in these circumstances. Thuja is a valuable remedy when there are no good indications for anything else in cases of acute bronchitis, slow to clear up, as pointed out by Clarke. If the patient has had a bad reaction to vaccination and/or a shiny face, these are excellent confirmatory symptoms.

Drosera is probably a better routine prescription for the aftermath of whooping cough than Pertussin. Drosera, being a proved remedy, may be symptomatically indicated, but often the choice is virtually impossible. Pertussin can be tried later if Drosera does not work.

A woman of 37 had suffered from migraine since childhood. The headaches were accompanied by an opening and shutting sensation in the head. After two years of prescribing she had fewer and less severe headaches. She was difficult, as there were too many 'good prescribing symptoms'. Then one day she complained of a cough, which on enquiry was found to be paroxysmal, and she had had bouts of paroxysmal coughing lasting a few days every year since whooping cough at the age of eight. She did not know whether or not whooping cough had preceded the migraine attacks, which maybe was not important in any case. Drosera 200c, lM and 10M was given. It had to be repeated six months later, since when she has been almost completely free from migraine for three years.

A woman of 38 complained of 'rheumatism of the left shoulder'. There was some wasting of the muscles of the shoulder girdle, which followed poliomyelitis eight years previously. Arsenicum Alb. 200c, t.i.d. 2 days, b.d. 2 days, was prescribed. She was unduly weak, worse at midnight, chilly and had burning pains relieved by warmth. The treatment worked like a charm, but the pains returned immediately it was stopped. A second course was given with nearly as good a result, then a higher potency was given, but with not much effect. Lathyrus Sativa 1M, three doses 12 hourly, was given and the pains cleared up for six months, when Lathyrus Sativa 1M was again prescribed. She had no further pain for about 3½ years, when again Lathyrus was followed by relief.

It does not seem to matter how long after a severe acute infection the appropriate remedy is given. Shortly after the war I was treating an elderly man for fibrositis of the lumbar region and troublesome paraesthesia of the lower limbs. Despite the fact that careful investigation failed to reveal anything serious, he did not respond to treatment at all until he received Typhoidinum 200c on account of typhoid fever he had had in 1886. The following month he came up saying he felt very much better. Glandular fever may be very slow to clear up. Carcinosin may be a useful remedy for such cases.

Pyrogen is sometimes useful when there is a history of septicaemia, severe after-effects of dental extraction, or ill-health commencing after an abortion in the absence of any obvious pelvic pathology. Enquiry should always be made, when possible, as to whether or not the mother suffered from any acute infection during pregnancy. The influence of German measles and probably other infections in causing malformation of the foetus has been established, and it is therefore likely that less obvious after-effects occur in the same way that post-natal illnesses may leave their mark.

Chronic Infection

Tuberculosis and venereal disease may call for the appropriate nosode, but fortunately these nosodes have been well proved and thoroughly clinically tested. It would be only in the absence of response to other apparently indicated remedies that they should be prescribed on the basis of the history alone.

The therapeutic field of nosodes of infection is vast and probably important, thought not easy to exploit with our present limited knowledge. For example, brucellosis, with its protean manifestations, often missed because it is not considered as a diagnostic possibility, is regarded by some authorities as a widespread infection in the UK. There is practically no reference to brucellosis in the homoeopathic literature at all.

Nosodes tend to be neglected in homoeopathic practice because of the influence of Hahnemann's theory of chronic disease and Kent's powerful endorsement of much of it.

Injury

Arnica montana has been used domestically for centuries for the effects of falls and bruises, and its proving demonstrated that Arnica acts homoeopathically. Arnica has been extensively used in homoeopathic practice throughout the world for generations as the first remedy for the after-effects of injury. In any condition which has resulted from an injury, Arnica is worthy of consideration when other remedies fail, and is the remedy of choice when there are no special indications for another remedy.

For the after-effects of head injury there are a group of remedies, Arnica, Cicuta, Hypericum, Natrum Mur., Natrum Sulph. and Helleborus, and these demand consideration also if there is a history of difficult birth. A child of six years of age took cold very frequently, had never thrived properly. He was markedly underweight, and had 'no interest in life', very sensitive to noise, afraid of the noise of a high wind and had other symptoms of Natrum Sulph. The history of a difficult birth confirmed the choice and the adminstration of Natrum Sulph. was followed by a rapid improvement in health, both mentally and physically.

Occasionally patients react in other ways after head injury. One child developed Nux Vomica symptoms and was helped by Nux Vomica. The list of such remedies is merely a record of frequent clinical associations.

Hypericum is the main remedy for spinal injuries. A woman of 34 developed ulcerative colitis which she attributed to a fall in which she hurt her back nine months previously. Her constitutional remedy was Sepia, which she was given with some benefit, although not as much as one would expect. Higher potencies were given, as the indications for Sepia seemed absolutely clear, but the results were not satisfactory. On the family history and the complementary relationship between Sepia and Carcinosin, a dose of Carcinosin 200c was then given, but again without any dramatic effect. Hypericum 30c, 200c, 1M on consecutive days was given and a month later she said 'I'm cured'. There was a slight relapse two months later for which Hypericum was given, and she has been well for over a year. This is the kind of case which makes one feel that it is sometimes necessary to directly antidote some episode of the past.

Another woman of 45 suffered from ulcerative colitis for several years. I treated her for about three years with fair results, till she was given a high potency of Arnica on account of an old severe injury. She has been remarkably better during the past two years.

Everyone has been injured at some time or another; it is only when there has been an injury in relation to the onset of ill-health, or when there has been a severe injury in the past, that it should call for consideration in constitutional prescribing.

Psychic Factors
Sometimes there is a clear history of a complaint starting after grief, fear or other emotional upset. The lists of remedies clinically associated with such precipitating causes found in Kent's *Repertory* and elsewhere may be valuable in giving confirmation to an individually chosen remedy. A boy of 15 years had suffered from enuresis since the age of 2½. He had been dry at 18 months but reverted to bedwetting when his mother was admitted to hospital. Many treatments had been given in vain before he came to homoeopathy. The boy was grossly overweight and had other

symptoms suggesting Graphites, which is one of the remedies known to have the 'effects of grief'. He was given Graphites CM. There was an aggravation for a week or so then a remission for some months, when he had a slight recurrence. Graphites CM was given again and he has been free from bedwetting for over a year. Of course, he might have 'grown out of it', but the case illustrates the way in which knowledge of the precipitating cause may help to confirm the choice of a remedy.

Many years ago I saw an excellent example of the use of Opium for the effects of fright, or to be more accurate, the value of Opium for a patient who reacted to fright in the Opium way. A woman developed exophthalmic goitre which came on suddenly after a severe fright. Dr Tyler elicited the characteristic Opium fear symptom, which is that when the frightening incident is recalled, the patient experiences fear long after, maybe months or, in this case, years after. Opium CM cured her.

Very occasionally Opium is useful post-operatively, when an old fright is presumably restimulated by another frightening experience. A boy of eleven was extremely ill, for no obvious reason, after an operation designed to reconstruct a badly injured shoulder. On the strength of this possibility I gave Opium CM and the remedy had a very beneficial effect. A boy of six developed a temperature of 39.5°C after removal of tonsils and adenoids. A course of antibiotics was given by the house surgeon but the temperature was unaffected. I saw the boy, and prescribed Sulphur 200c on 'absence of prescribing symptoms', again without result. Then on re-examining him in case something had been missed, my attention was drawn to a large burn scar on his abdomen. There was nothing else to go on and I prescribed Opium CM. This was followed by a drop in temperature overnight. Afterwards I questioned the mother, who said that the boy had screamed every time anyone touched his tummy from the time of the burn at 18 months till he was three years old – a typical Opium symptom.

Quite often other remedies are of course required for the after-effects of fright. A girl of nine developed psoriasis in the form of small rounded areas less than a centimetre in diameter after a fright. Opium CM was prescribed over the telephone but without any apparent benefit. When the mother brought the girl to see me it was obvious that in this case the remedy was Aurum Met., which also has 'the effects of fright'. It was given in the 200c potency. This was followed by an aggravation, then the psoriasis cleared up for a few months, but returned. Aurum Met. 10M was prescribed and the psoriasis disappeared and has not recurred during the past two years.

A girl of 3½ years was admitted to hospital with a temperature of

40.5°C in a drowsy delirious state. Her blood count showed 38,000 W.B.C., mainly polymorphs. The only positive finding on clinical examination was evidence of sinusitis accompanied by large tender cervical glands. The child was dangerously ill. Her face was hot and flushed. The pupils were pinpoint. She was muttering about 'flies' although there were none in the ward and she was obviously frightened, but not from any apparent external cause. I ordered an antibiotic and Opium CM to be given hourly at first. That was 1.30 p.m. At 4.30 p.m. she was sitting on her mother's lap watching television. The temperature had fallen to 39°C and by 8.30 p.m. that evening the temperature was 37°C. There was a slight return of fever the next day which subsided the following day, and the blood count came down dramatically. She made an uneventful recovery. The antibiotic had not been given and was never needed. The cause of such a high temperature and much raised white blood count was never satisfactorily explained. On questioning the mother, she said that her child had been frightened by a wasp three weeks before, which might conceivably have explained the 'flies', but one cannot be sure. However, she was apparently 'stuck in fright', which is another way of describing the Opium fear reaction.

Sometimes an emotional upset may apparently occur prenatally. A girl of sixteen was slow in recovering from influenza. Thinking back over the twelve years I had looked after her, this was the usual pattern; there was sluggishness in recovering from every acute illness for no obvious reason. Going back over the history I discovered that the mother had been frightened by a doctor during pregnancy on being told that she might lose her baby. She said, 'I felt the shock go right through me.' The girl was given Opium CM and made a quicker recovery, but not only that, she became physically more robust and her ability to study increased quite definitely.

Staphysagria is well known for its effects when there is a strong sense of injustice. A number of remedies have this – listed in Kent's repertory under 'Mortification' – but Staphysagria is most often needed when this is a leading symptom, in my experience.

As a rule children greatly prefer to be in the ward with other children rather than in a cubicle. One little boy, however, objected strongly when he was admitted to the general ward. Everything was wrong, and he insisted he be put back in his cubicle. The ward sister detected a strong sense of injustice and gave him a dose of Staphysagria 200c. She told me that within ten minutes he was delighted to be in the ward and everything was fine! Sometimes there is a prolonged feeling of injustice. Dr Tyler quoted a very typical case of an army officer who had been passed over as regards promotion during the First World War and came back into civilian life generally unwell and disgruntled. He was given Staphysagria in high potency with excellent results.

Causticum is sometimes indicated after acute fright or prolonged anxiety. In 1939 a man of 52 came to the hospital suffering from loss of voice. He was distressed because he was the foreman of a factory which was closing down and he had to give notice to his men, some well on in years, who might find difficulty in getting other work. Causticum is worth trying for loss of voice whether from psychological or inflammatory causes, when there is little on which to prescribe accurately. Additionally, it covered the man's sympathetic nature. The interesting thing about him was that he had been buried alive during the First World War, and when rescued it was discovered that his hair had fallen out. He had been almost completely bald since 1916. He was given Causticum 200c and his voice returned soon after. About two months later he said that his wife and daughter had noticed that his hair was growing in. A fine downy fluff, about a quarter of an inch in depth, covered the bald patch. I saw him after the war and there was no further growth of hair, even with higher potencies of Causticum and other remedies. The remarkable feature was that Causticum apparently had caused such an effect after twenty-three years.

DRUGS

Hahnemann observed that Nux Vomica was a useful remedy for 'the evil consequences of coffee and wine drinking' and since then Nux Vomica has been extensively used for the after-effects of drugs in general. Pulsatilla has been found effective in treating patients upset by iron. Natrum Mur. and other remedies have been used to counteract the effects of prolonged drugging with quinine in malarious districts.

Thus certain relationships have been established between constitution and the influence of drugs. As a rule, constitutional treatment can deal with the after-effects of drugs once the drug has been excreted. There are also many records of drug effects being antidoted by the same drug given in potency. It is better to prescribe constitutionally first, as a potency of the drug may either work dramatically or not at all. It is interesting that the same applies to the nosodes of acute infection in respect of ill-health following an acute illness, as already mentioned.

Dr Charles C. Bowes related a case in which a potency of the chemical responsible for the illness was successful in curing. 'A child of four years falling into short spells of unconsciousness, unable to control the flow of urine day or night, was absolutely cured by a dose of Terebinthina 1M. The history of the case was that the child had drunk a lot of turpentine when 18 months old and had gone from bad to worse ever since. She never had a fit after that dose, and gradually but quickly got over the enuresis.'

Some years ago I treated a child suffering from an almost purely allergic type of asthma. The attacks occurred about once a week on an average. The first attack had been apparently caused by inhaling sulphur fumes. In this case the constitutional remedy was Sulphur, which was given in the 30th, later the 200th, potency at long intervals, repeating when there was a relapse. The child was completely cured.

A woman of forty-two developed psoriasis consisting of rounded areas about 2 centimetres in diameter, widely distributed over her trunk and limbs, after treatment for tonsillitis with sulphapyridine. Arsenicum Alb. was prescribed but without any effect, and a month later she was given Sulphapyridine 30c. The psoriasis cleared up completely and had not returned six years later. Many cases of this kind have been reported in the homoeopathic literature in respect of a wide range of chemicals.

Sometimes the child may be affected by drugs taken by the mother. In another case previously recorded, a boy of fourteen was said by his teachers to be intelligent, but somehow 'could not use his brain'. His mother had been taking pethidine during pregnancy on account of osteomyelitis. The boy was given Pethidine 30c and his ability to study shot up.

It is interesting to speculate on what exactly happens in such cases, when the drug which has adversely influenced a patient helps drama- tically when given in potency. Is it that in these successful cases the drug is in fact one of the constitutional remedies for that individual, that it would have helped in any case, whether or not the patient had had an overdose of it?

For some years now I have taken the 'anaesthetic history' of every patient and this is occasionally very rewarding in constitutional pre- scribing. The most definite feature which has emerged is that patients suffering from liver or gallbladder disease, who have had a bad reaction to chloroform, usually benefit from chloroform in potency. Such a history is often obtainable from older patients. It is probable that this just means that chloroform, with its known toxic effect on the liver, may be a useful 'pathological' liver remedy.

An infant of six months kept her parents awake through flatulence although there was no obvious feeding mismanagement. Lycopodium and Raphanus were helpful, but the parents were getting worn out through lack of sleep despite this. The child had been born by caesarean section in 1961, and it is very unlikely that any chloroform was given. As there was a possibility of some very slight liver damage I tried Chloroform 30c, and there has been no trouble for the past nine months.

A man of forty-five who had suffered from very severe attacks of asthma for ten years responded to some extent to constitutional treatment. He had been born under chloroform anaesthesia, and his mother had been greatly upset by the anaesthetic. Natrum Sulph. and Lachesis, both liver remedies, had seemed to help him. He was given Chloroform 30c, and later 200c, and has been practically free from asthma for over three years.

A woman of twenty complained of bouts of colicky epigastric pains which began at the age of eight. The attacks had become much more frequent and more severe during the previous year. Investigations were all negative. Colocynth 3x was found to be an effective remedy in relieving the pains, but despite careful constitutional treatment the number of attacks, about one in two weeks, was not reduced. There was a strong family history of cancer and four siblings had been helped by Carcinosin. Carcinosin Adeno. Stom. 30c was given, but without apparent effect. She was the only one of the family born under chloroform anaesthesia and on this fact, together with symptoms of liver dysfunction, Chloroform 30c was tried. The attacks cleared for three months and then returned, but not so severely. Chloroform 100c was given and followed by practically complete freedom for over three years. She became pregnant, and during the pregnancy the colicky pains returned quite severely. She came to see me and Chloroform 200c wiped out the pains.

OTHER FACTORS

A number of items may be of value in some cases. Exposure to radiation, if judged to be excessive, may call for a trial of X-ray 30c or 200c or Radium Bromide 30c or 200c as intercurrent remedies. Illnesses beginning at puberty suggest a careful look at Pulsatilla, and when ill-health starts after the menopause, Lachesis and others.

FAMILY HISTORY

In making a psychomatic homoeopathic prescription or a prescription based on the individual's past history, the patient is regarded against a background of a theoretical norm. The same applies to 'family history' and the same rule regarding any uncertain symptoms – if in doubt discard them and look for something definite. Should there be a strong history of tuberculosis or cancer in the family, the appropriate nosodes deserve consideration. Recent studies of Carcinosin suggest that it may be a useful remedy when one or more of the following group of diseases are strongly represented in the family history: carcinoma, leukaemia, tuberculosis and diabetes.

Chapter 6

Homoeopathic Prescribing in Childhood

The selection of a homoeopathic remedy in childhood is made in the same way as in adults. The difference lies mainly in case-taking and in interpreting the symptoms against the normal pattern of behaviour at any particular age.

The history is supplied to greater or lesser extent by the mother or nurse, at any rate by someone other than the patient himself.

In formulating a plan of case-taking it is therefore necessary to concentrate on symptoms which can readily be observed by someone other than the patient. The mother is usually by far the best person to give the history, especially when the patient is an infant.

Not only is the mother a keen observer of her infant, but she can often give us an account of the family history, and a first-hand account of the period of gestation and labour.

Intra-uterine Environmental Factors
The discovery that German measles in the mother can produce deformity in the foetus has focused attention on this important part of the child's life. Microcephaly, congenital heart disease, cataract and deafness are the most common abnormalities.

The period of most danger to the foetus is during the early months of gestation. Studies have indicated that when the mother became infected during the first two months of pregnancy the chances of foetal deformity were 100 per cent. In the third month the figure dropped to 50 per cent. Viruses can readily pass through the placenta. In the influenza epidemic of 1918 a high proportion of infected mothers aborted. It is well known that syphilis and occasionally other infections may be transmitted to the foetus, causing injury or death.

The use of lead as an abortifacient can cause foetal abnormalities, especially congenital heart disease and skeletal defects. The therapeutic use of X-rays and radium can cause foetal defects, especially microcephaly.

Dennis Browne has demonstrated how intra-uterine pressure can cause talipes and other deformities.

If there were any doubt that the foetus can be adversely affected by its environment in utero there are instances recorded of deformity of one of similar twins.

Dr Landtman of University College Hospital, London, sums up as follows: 'Various observations have shown that environmental principles play an important part in the aetiology of congenital malformations. Foetal abnormalities result, but not of any characteristic type in relation to the various causes. The most important factor appears to be the stage at which foetal development is disturbed. Due to lack of teratogenetic characteristics, malformations caused by environmental agents may simulate abnormalities of genetic origin.'

Drugs taken by the mother can undoubtedly affect the foetus in some cases. All textbooks on obstetrics condemn the use of alcohol during and immediately after pregnancy, suggesting it as a possible cause of sterility, abortion, still-birth and a high foetal mortality.

There is experimental evidence that alcohol tends to concentrate in the reproductive organs, and it is freely diffusible through the placenta. Carpenter has shown that in hens with immature eggs that were exposed to the fumes of alcohol for periods of two to twenty-nine hours, the concentration of alcohol in the egg was often equal to or greater than the concentration in the bloodstream.

The evidence about smoking during pregnancy indicates that it will affect the foetus. The effect of nicotine in breast milk is referred to later.

The placenta is also permeable to chloroform, ether, morphia, hyoscine, atropine, physostigmine, pilocarpine, arsphenamine, the barbiturates, sulphonamides, penicillin and various salts of sodium, potassium, copper and bismuth.

Marked emotional disturbance may affect the unborn child, and no homoeopathic history is complete without a record of any such episodes.

The Effects of Labour

In the process of birth the infant is exposed to trauma of varying degree, to anoxia, and sometimes to anaesthetics.

These observations have been made as a reminder of environmental influences before or during birth, rather than to stress unduly the risks encountered by the foetus during gestation and labour. Occasionally some outstanding event of pregnancy or labour is of the utmost value in prescribing.

It is obvious that we should consider specially the events of pregnancy and labour in children who have never thrived. Faulty milk teeth also suggests an enquiry into pregnancy, as these teeth are formed in the second half of gestation. It is, of course, impossible to rule out hereditary influences in this connection.

The Home Environment in Relation to Symptoms

Even in infancy, children are acutely aware of the mental atmosphere of the home or the people around them. The nervous child has almost inevitably been brought up in an atmosphere of fear and worry. The effects of a 'broken home', where father and mother have separated or are mentally incompatible, are highly damaging. It has been noticed in child guidance clinics that the 'broken home' is a frequent cause of juvenile delinquency. One of the basic needs of childhood is a sense of emotional security. In the 'broken home' he does not feel secure. When a young child, under the age of five years, is removed from his mother for a period of six months or longer, there is statistical evidence to show that this child has a greater tendency to develop into a juvenile delinquent than average.

Almost equally damaging to the child is a feeling of insecurity engendered by ambitious parents who make the child feel he is valued for his achievements rather than for himself.

If it is forgotten that children tend to react in a similar way to their mental environment, mental symptoms may be evaluated too highly, as being characteristic of the individual. Also in such cases the environment may be too strong for the child to overcome, even if the correct homoeopathic treatment is given.

Feeding in Relation to Symptoms

Infant feeding is now well supervised although mistakes still occur, and in infancy the amount and nature of the feeds should be ascertained. The technique of feeding must also be considered carefully. If this is overlooked, symptoms arising from mismanagement may easily be mistaken for constitutional ones.

We have to remember the possibility of contamination of food, and this applies to breast milk too. Many drugs are excreted in the milk but adverse effects on the infant are few. Nicotine is excreted in the milk of mothers who smoke during lactation. Moderate smoking (up to seven cigarettes per day) appears to have no ill effects on the breast-fed infant. The amount of nicotine excreted in the milk in mothers who smoke over fifteen cigarettes per day is considered potentially harmful to the infant. Dr W. H. Thompson, writing in the *American Journal of Obstetrics and*

Gynecology states, 'When one considers the statements of Cushney that nicotine is about as poisonous as prussic acid, it seems logical to consider that even minute quantities of nicotine administered through breast milk might upset digestive processes to the extent of endangering the early growth of delicate babies.'

The preparation of food in aluminium pans may cause harm. Copper cooking utensils are much less widely used. They can cause symptoms if not kept clean. Many babies of mothers who smoke or use drugs, and many children fed on food cooked in aluminium seem perfectly well. It seems to be largely a matter of sensitivity whether the individual suffers or not, particularly when only small amounts of toxins are ingested.

Post-natal History
The mother can usually supply us with an accurate list of acute illness, reaction to immunisation, trauma, mental or physical, and any drugs given to the child in chronological order. The mother usually gives some valuable clues to the nature of the child, in addition to what we can observe for ourselves. It is useful, however, to have some plan of interrogation in mind, based on the symptoms of high value which the mother is in a position to observe.

Generalities with Special Reference to Childhood
From earliest infancy there are signs of individuality. The infant spends most of its time in feeding and sleeping. Observation in any children's ward will show that during sleep many children tend to take up characteristic positions. A large proportion of children do so during the first year. In many children the tendency disappears or may alter later. In some it persists. Kent's *Repertory* lists only one remedy for the knee-elbow position, 'Sleep position, on the knees with face forced into the pillow', Medorrhinum. Enquiry of the position adopted in sleep suggests that Lycopodium or Sepia, Tuberculinum, Calc. Phos. and probably other remedies also have this symptom. The value of it is that the mother can usually give a definite answer to the question and it is obviously a generality.

Occasionally, the infant's response to being picked up and especially to being laid down may be useful. Aversion to downward motion, as when the baby is laid down in its cot, may confirm the selection of Borax.

Enquiry into sleep and dreams may be of value. The older child can relate his dreams. Night terrors are often caused through mechanical blockage of the air passage by enlarged tonsils and adenoids. In these circumstances night terrors are obviously not of high value in prescribing.

48

As regards food, very young infants may show marked preference for warm feeds. They will staunchly refuse a bottle which has been chilled. Others do not mind, and a few have a distinct preference for cold feeds.

At the stage of weaning, it is customary for the infant to reject its first mouthful of a new food, for example yolk of egg, and if the mother does not persist this might be mistaken for an aversion. In any case it is probable that we are on less firm ground with aversions than with cravings. Children are easily put off by example or suggestion, or possibly by being compelled to eat any article of diet when not hungry. Forcing children to eat not only causes mental tension at the dining table, but may change indifference into a positive dislike of any particular food.

It is very rare for the mother's milk to upset a child. The most common fault is that it may be insufficient. This can readily be ascertained by test weighing.

In questioning the mother about cravings or aversions to food it is useful to keep in mind the following list:

    Cow: meat, fat, milk, butter, cheese, ice-cream.
    Pig: bacon, bacon fat, bacon rind.
    Fish
    Eggs
    Potatoes
    Other vegetables
    Fruit
    Bread
    Sweets
    Salt, pepper, vinegar.

Naturally a desire for ice-cream or sweets is not accepted unless it is very strong in childhood. Aversion to sweets is a peculiar symptom.

It is surprising how many children have a craving for bacon fat or rind. (Calc. Phos., Tuberculinum) Some children love eating bacon rind raw.

Craving for salt or vinegar are not uncommon in childhood. The mother may have to keep the salt cellar or vinegar bottle out of reach.

A boy of two months was sent by a welfare clinic to the outpatients' department. His mother said he took his feeds well, but vomited if he took very much. He cried all day but slept well at night. He was put on artificial food at the age of one week. Three attempts had been made at the welfare centre to get him on the right diet, without success. He was now on a well-balanced diet of fresh cow's milk, sugar and water.

The baby looked ill, his skin was dry, his forehead wrinkled, and the anterior fontenelle slightly depressed. Nothing else was noted on clinical examination. The mantoux was negative; urine negative. He was very much under-weight. His birth weight was 8lb. 10oz. Instead of gaining two or three pounds he had only gained two ounces.

On enquiry from the mother and father the following facts were elicited. He was most miserable between 4 and 9 p.m. He refused feeds if they were the least bit cool. He invariably slept in the knee-elbow position. He was given Medorrhinum and later Lycopodium. He gained one pound in the first sixteen days after commencing treatment. His mother was advised to gradually increase the feeds. By the end of two months he was 'very happy' and his mother noted that he now lay on his side for the first time. He was followed up for five months. He was then seven months old, weighed 16lb., and was cutting his first teeth.

This case is given to illustrate the symptoms of high value which can be observed by the parents.

The mental make-up of a child may express itself quite clearly from infancy. Some babies are irritable, others placid and so on. Sensitivity to noise is common in young babies, so unless the baby 'nearly jumps out of its skin' at slight noises it may safely be disregarded as an individual characteristic.

In asking the mother about her child's disposition a number of symptoms can be associated with the words 'affection' and 'sympathy'. It is normal for babies and children to require affection, but it is strongly marked in some, and in others a desire for affection may show itself only in association with an acute illness. Some babies from the earliest days dislike to be picked up. Some children have a tendency to become indifferent to their parents, which is a valuable symptom when there is no apparent reason for it, suggesting Sepia or Phosphorus, etc. The mother can almost always speak quite definitely on this subject. Is the child sympathetic to others; concerned with the troubles of others outside the family circle, or to cruelty? Occasionally there is a cruel streak in the child.

It is sometimes difficult to decide whether a childish fear is inherent or implanted by suggestion. If you protect a young child from the affectionate onslaught of a puppy, fear may be created in the child's mind. In a nervous child with nervous parents, fear of dogs would not have the same significance as it would in a mentally more stable child. When in doubt it is as well to discard a fear which may have been created by suggestion, and look instead for other symptoms of high value such as a craving for salt or other general symptoms. When discussing fears it is, of course, advisable to speak to the mother in the absence of the child. It is as well to keep in mind that very young children often understand much more than we are apt to think. A normal child in its second year understands a considerable amount of what is said in simple language.

The fondness for dancing which is a characteristic of Sepia is sometimes manifest in childhood. But it is the rule rather than the exception for young children to 'dance' on hearing music. A boy of twelve suffering from second stage nephritis had been attending the outpatients' department for some years with only slight improvement. Symptoms such as 'indifference to loved ones' suggested Sepia. When the mother was asked about dancing she said, 'Oh, he is crazy about dancing'. At this age it is an unusual symptom. He was given Sepia 200c, which was followed by a marked improvement in his general health and appearance.

Jealousy is not uncommon in childhood. Most often the first child is jealous of a new arrival. The normal child is untidy, but an extreme tendency in this respect often confirmed by the child's appearance strongly suggests Sulphur, especially if the child just cannot be kept clean. On the other hand, the fastidious child will put his toys away neatly in rows without being asked. On enquiring of a mother if her little girl of four was unduly tidy, she replied, 'Tidy, yes. She even keeps me tidy too.' Needless to say, Arsenicum Alb. and Nux Vomica are to be considered when this symptom is present. 'Desire for travel' must be marked before it can be accepted as an individual characteristic in childhood.

We must consider the child's reaction to its physical environment – heat, cold, wet weather, thundery weather, stuffy rooms, sea air, etc., as in the case of adults.

The combination of amelioration at the seaside, and adoption of the knee-elbow position in sleep (Medorrhinum), is not infrequently met with in asthmatic children. In assessing our results in asthma it is important to keep in mind that four out of five asthmatic children recover as they grow older, without any treatment. Time modalities can be observed in the youngest infant. It should not be forgotten that many young children become tired and 'grizzly' towards bedtime.

Finally, the mother can observe any skin symptoms, such as perspiration, its odour and, if localised, its distribution, on the head or feet for example. Skin eruptions of any sort are easily noted by the mother.

The Prescription

The most accurate method of remedy selection is by comparison of the individual symptom of the patient with remedy provings.

In cases where the illness began during gestation, there is often some striking episode which is vividly remembered by the mother, most commonly a fright or an acute virus infection. In such cases we can sometimes distinguish between Aconite, Ignatia, Opium, Natrum Mur. or other suggested remedies. In the case of an acute infection the symptoms may not be sufficiently clear and the use of an unproved nosode is justified.

In childhood, ill-health may date from an acute infection such as pneumonia, from vaccination or immunisation against diphtheria. There seem to be more cases of ill-health after immunisation than after vaccination at present. In addition to the accurate selection of a remedy from the totality of symptoms we may use the appropriate nosode, such as Pneumococcin, Morbillinum, Parotidinum or Diphtherinum, when the apparently indicated remedy fails. Sometimes the effect is magical, at other times little or no effect is obtained. The reason for this is not clear. It may be that these nosodes have a very limited sphere of action, or it may be that the nosode and patient are in different electro-physical groups. Whatever the reason for failure in some cases these nosodes are too valuable to discard on any theoretical grounds. The nosodes of acute infections are specially valuable when there is a history of severe or prolonged acute illness, and above all when this occurred in the first or second year of life.

Through the works of Bach, Wheeler and Paterson, a new approach to remedy selection has opened up. There is a mass of experimental evidence to show that the intestinal flora is related to the health of an individual and that the bowel flora can be altered by potentised drugs. Guidance in selection of the remedy may be obtained from stool analysis of non-lactose fermenting organisms. From a study of the symptomatology associated with specific states of the intestinal flora, remedy pictures have been evolved. The bowel nosodes are specially valuable in childhood. Morgan Co., and Morgan Pure (Paterson) are the 'skin nosodes' and are often required in infantile eczema. Dysentery Co., has a specific action on the pylorus, and has a clinical record in pylorospasm and in congenital pyloric stenosis.

The association of remedies with pathological states is helpful in prescribing in childhood as in other fields of medicine. The use of Arnica for the infant (and the mother) after difficult labour, Alumina for constipation in breast-fed infants and Chamomilla in painful dentition are well-known examples.

For over forty years Lathyrus Sativa has been widely used as an effective prophylactic in infantile paralysis. Diphtherinum 200c has proved a successful safeguard against diphtheria in an epidemic or when given to contacts. Dr Paterson has demonstrated that Diphtherinum in potency can alter the Schick reaction from negative to positive. The association of various remedies with the acute infections of childhood is well-known. Dr Burnett's 'specific' for mumps was Pilocarpine Muriate 3x. Either the salt or Pilocarpine itself in 30th potency seems to have an almost specific effect in mumps. There is one skin condition of childhood which is definitely associated with a remedy – impetigo contagiosa and Antimony. Dr Tyler's 'specific' was Antimonium Tart.

Pneumonia, which strikes hardest at the extremes of life, is admirably studied from the viewpoint of associated remedies by Dr Borland. His booklet *Pneumonias* is an invaluable guide.

Finally, there is the Down's syndrome child. Nothing can be done to alter the genetic characteristics, but almost invariably these children are helped physically and mentally by Medorrhinum.

Chapter 7

Paediatric Case-Taking

One of the reasons why there is a reluctance to get to grips with case-taking is that Hahnemann's theory of chronic disease is at present neither fully accepted nor completely rejected, and there is no alternative comprehensive theory to replace it. Every experienced homoeopath recognises in his patients the images of Hahnemann's Psora, Sycosis and Syphilis, but as a rule not so accurately or consistently that this can be made the basis of his everyday practice. It is, however, generally agreed that the aim of homoeopathic treatment of chronic ill-health, apart from dealing with the end results of disease, is to treat the patient. The difference between an ordinary medical history and a 'homoeopathic' history is that the object of the former is to serve as a pointer to the pathological diagnosis, whereas the latter extends beyond this and includes information about the patient which may be utilised in the selection of similar remedies. The place of homoeopathy or other forms of treatment can best be assessed from the pathological diagnosis, but the application of homoeopathic treatment depends on a careful appraisal of the individual patient, on what might be termed a 'diagnosis of the patient'.

Special Features of Paediatric Case-taking
The chief difference between paediatric case-taking and that of older age groups is that the patient has to be regarded against a background of a norm which not only differs from the adult norm, but changes considerably from infancy to puberty. The mother, or someone with an intimate knowledge of the child, is the best person to give the history in infancy and early childhood. Even up to puberty the child does not readily look at himself objectively. An obvious advantage of having the mother is that she is able to give an account of the family history, has first-hand knowledge of pregnancy and labour, and has usually been in a position to observe any outstanding episodes in the child's early life, such as a severe reaction to vaccination, injury, severe acute infection or an

emotional upset. This does not mean to imply that the older child's evidence should be discarded, but even in apparently obvious things such as cravings or aversions to foods, the mother can usually give more accurate information.

The Mother's History
The mother should be allowed to tell the story in her own way without interruption, just as she might give her own history. Only in this way may certain invaluable clues be disclosed which might otherwise be lost. The emphasis given by the mother to various symptoms is noted in the same way that an adult history is appropriately underlined. The importance of obtaining really definite symptoms cannot be stressed too strongly.

Dr Tyler used to say in regard to homoeopathic case-taking that the longer she lived the less she wrote down. The homoeopathic materia medica is so vast, and there is so much overlapping, that the best way to accurate prescribing is to select really definite symptoms characteristic of the individual; one of the remedies which adequately covers these is likely to cover the rest of the case.

Classification of Constitutional Remedies
It is useful to keep in mind a rough classification of the ways in which similar remedies are used in constitutional treatment. I think of these as comprising three overlapping groups:
1) Remedies prescribed on the basis of a similarity between the psychosomatic make-up of the patient and the drug picture, such as Sepia or Sulphur.
2) Remedies administered with the object of antidoting some adverse influence of the past, including family history, the period of gestation, labour, and outstanding post-natal events.
3) 'Pathological', etc. This group comprises pathological remedies, the bowel nosodes, autogenous potencies, sarcodes, hormones, and vitamins. In history-taking we are mainly concerned with the first two groups.

Generals and Particulars
Whilst making a note of the history it is necessary to clearly separate symptoms pertaining to the patient, such as a craving for ice-cream or a tendency to sweaty feet, from those relating to the illness. If a child suffers from asthma, the group of symptoms relating to an acute attack must be kept separate from the symptoms reflecting the psychosomatic make-up of the patient. A remedy which covers the attack will abort it,

but no matter how often the attacks are cured, the tendency to have them is unaltered until the patient himself is treated constitutionally.

Interrogation of the Mother
The mother's history is clarified by questions on points she has raised, such as how definite a symptom is, and whether it can be taken to be outside the average pattern or not; if not, it is discarded as a repertorising symptom. Next, the picture is filled in by systematic questioning, and here arises a problem. Too long a list of questions leads to boredom and failure to achieve its ends, and too short a one could omit important symptoms and also end in failure. Whatever plan of questioning is adopted, it can only be effective with a background of knowledge of the materia medica.

If the following four headings are kept in mind – 'Foods', 'Environment', 'Mentals', and the 'Serial History' – sufficient information on which to base prescriptions will almost always be found.

Repertorisation
From the first three, the salient psychosomatic features of the patient can be delineated, and Dr Leon Vannier has pointed out that the most valuable and certainly the most useful symptoms on which to repertorise are those which he terms 'entrusted characteristics of the individual'. That is to say, symptoms which are not apparently related to hereditary or environmental influences. For instance, a craving for salt in a child whose siblings do not crave it, or a sensitivity to music in one child of an unmusical family, can be taken as an 'entrusted characteristic'. While it might be difficult or impossible to prove that neither hereditary nor environmental influences played a part in its causation, it is nevertheless an invaluable criterion to the selection of symptoms for repertorisation.

In dealing with the four symptom groups, only really definite symptoms should be taken and then they must be considered against what is normal for a child of the same age group.

Rather than deal with every detail, a selection of some of the main symptoms are considered here, with the object of pointing out the way in which symptoms are evaluated.

Foods
The mother should be given to understand clearly that what we are after is information about any definite cravings or aversions to food or drink. It is wise to run through a list of foods rapidly, so that she may pick on one or more items which stand out; otherwise she may waste time trying to be precise about irrelevant details.

These symptoms must be appraised against the norm. An aversion to sweets is of more value than a desire for sweets, unless the latter is a craving outside the normal child's liking for sweets. Quite a few children eat salt by itself, and to be quite definite a 'desire for salt' should include this.

A desire for fat meat is unusual, and therefore all the more valuable if present. Most children like ice-cream and it is only outside the average pattern when a child is constantly asking for it.

Bottle-fed infants usually like their feeds lukewarm, but occasionally an infant refuses the bottle till it is cold, or another may refuse it if it gets the least bit chilled. If present, these are useful symptoms at an age when guides to constitution may be difficult to discover.

It is worthwhile to ask about bacon rind. The children who crave it are usually covered by Calc. Phos., Tuberculinum or Carcinosin. For children constantly drinking cold water, Tuberculinum should be considered first.

Sometimes an aversion to food is natural to a child; few children like onions, for instance. Sometimes an aversion may be conditioned. If father cuts the fat off his meat, a child might copy him.

Aluminium Cooking Utensils

It is my practice to advise their discontinuance in certain circumstances. Sometimes when taking the history, symptoms corresponding to the provings of Aluminium come out strongly. If not, the answer to three questions can usually provide information which may suggest looking into the subject further. Children who are sensitive to aluminium usually exhibit two or three of the following symptoms easily noticed by the mother: (1) They tend to rub their eyes frequently; (2) There is straining at stool; (3) They are slow eaters.

The effects on eyelids are well known, also the weakness of the rectal muscles, and of the oesophagus. Occasionally in older children one gets the adult description of being conscious of a bolus of food going down. More often than not Aluminium is not the constitutional remedy; this may be Sepia, Lycopodium, or Carcinosin, etc., and I find that giving Alumina 200c, ten to fourteen days after the constitutional remedy seems to work very well.

Occasionally Alumina is the constitutional remedy. A girl of eleven years of age came with the complaint of leucorrhoea which had been investigated and treated by non-homoeopathic methods, but which kept returning. She had suffered also from headaches for three years, and alternating constipation and diarrhoea from the age of eighteen months.

This child had the triad of symptoms mentioned above and other Alumina symptoms. A change of cooking utensils, including the kettle, and a prescription of Alumina 200c was followed by a cessation of the leucorrhoea, headaches and bowel upset within a month. There was a slight return about six months later, when another prescription of Alumina 200c was followed by complete recovery for some months, after which she was not followed up.

It is probably worthwhile to stop aluminium in all allergic subjects. Sometimes school dinners provide a problem for less strong-minded parents. I use Alumina 30c, 200c or 1M as an antidote, given again when symptoms recur. Vitamin E 30c or 200c has in a few cases appeared also to be a very satisfactory antidote.

Environment
Under this heading we can ask about any unusual reaction, favourable or unfavourable, to the physical environment. Heat, cold, open air, sea air, sunshine, change of weather, windy weather, and thunderstorms.

Any outstanding symptoms such as 'Can't stand hot weather', or 'Always better at the seaside', or 'Always wants to be out in the open air', may be taken as a constitutional symptom.

A definite useful symptom is that complaints are better or worse in sea air. This means that a particular is raised to the value of a general because of its strength.

Probably all remedies influenced by sea are influenced both ways, although there may be a marked tendency in one direction. Natrum Mur. is about equally worse or better by the sea. Medorrhinum is almost always better, very rarely worse. The Tuberculinums are almost always worse, just occasionally better. Carcinosin has it both ways also, and is better at the East coast and worse in the South, or vice versa. In chilly patients it is worthwhile to find out if the patient is cold all over or only in parts, such as hands and feet, which suggests a sycotic remedy. Reaction to a thunderstorm may be an aggravation, fear, or enjoyment. Enjoys watching a storm is a useful confirmatory symptom of Sepia and Carcinosin. Fear has to be looked on against the family background, and the tendency for children to copy others.

It is convenient under the heading of environment to take into consideration events of the twenty-four hours, especially time modalities and sleep. If an infant gets 'grizzly' towards bedtime, that is not outside the normal pattern, but if the child is always worse at 10 a.m. (Natrum Mur.), 4-8 p.m. (Lycopodium usually), or 3-5 a.m. (Kali. Carb., etc.), for no apparent reason, this is worth noting.

In some cases it is only after failure to produce satisfactory results by apparently careful prescribing that a nightly aggravation is noticed. In such cases Lueticum is almost always indicated. Sometimes there is an aggravation after sleep which, of course, is not the same as a nightly aggravation. For example, asthma is often worse at night, but only occasionally does one get the history of 'attacks invariably commencing after sleep', in which cases Lachesis is often indicated.

Enquiry about sleep should not be omitted.

1) If insomnia is present, its type, e.g. lying awake late, may be useful as a confirmatory symptom.
2) Modalities of sleep, including effects of loss of sleep.
3) Appearance during sleep:
   (a) Position adopted. The knee-elbow position is common up to nine months or a year. After that it is much less often observed, so that its value as a symptom would be higher. The following remedies have it: Medorrhinum, Phosphorus, Calc. Phos., Tuberculinum, Sepia, Lycopodium and Carcinosin.
   (b) Perspiration and its distribution. A sweaty head at night is sometimes a useful confirmatory symptom for Calc. Phos.
   (c) Whether the child is restless, or kicks off the bedclothes.

Dreams in older children are not often helpful. Very occasionally there is a nightmare of this type. The child wakes up in terror, sometimes being afraid of something in the corner of the room, but after being reassured falls asleep and wakens in the morning without any knowledge of the episode. Phosphorus and Carcinosin have cured this condition. Dreams of falling are fairly common, and must be frequent if they are to be taken as having high value.

Mentals

It is probably better to leave mentals last, in case the mother thinks the doctor considers her child mentally abnormal, although, other things being equal, mental symptoms are of most importance. I usually start with 'affection', and ask if the child appears to want more affection than average or resent it ('consolation aggravates'). The average child needs affection, but if there is a craving for it, it is outside the usual pattern, whether or not it might have a psychological explanation. The child who never tires of affection often needs Pulsatilla, Phosphorus, a Phosphorus compound or Carcinosin. It is a valuable confirmatory symptom. Pulsatilla and Phosphorus differ in that Phosphorus is responsive and gives out affection, whereas Pulsatilla just absorbs it.

The next symptom one can enquire about is sympathy for others. This may be expressed quite early in life. Many children are most concerned if they think anyone is suffering, and if it is a concern over someone outside the family, such as being upset on hearing an unknown child cry, it is worthwhile taking it as a symptom. To the rubrics concerned with sympathy to others may be added Graphites, Sepia and Carcinosin.

Sensitivity to Music
The question is, does the child have an unusual appreciation of music? Some children show discrimination in their taste quite early, and this should not be confused with the average child's liking of music. It is unusual for a child not to like music, except when there is a sensitivity to noise and the radio is playing loudly. Most children have a sense of rhythm and jig about on hearing suitable tunes, but this is not synonymous with discrimination of taste. Down's syndrome and other mentally handicapped children usually have a keen appreciation of music, and in such patients it cannot therefore be taken as an individual symptom. A very strong sense of rhythm is a useful confirmatory symptom of Sepia and Carcinosin.

Obstinacy
The average child gradually begins to assert himself, but in some cases this takes the form of extreme obstinacy. If it is well outside the average assertiveness, it is a valuable symptom. The remedy to be first thought of for such children in Tub. Bov. 30c or higher. It might almost be said that the more obstinate the child, the more likely Tub. Bov. is indicated. On one occasion a child of six years had to be dragged into the out-patient consulting room loudly protesting. It was impossible to examine him, but from the history it seemed that he had chronic upper respiratory tract infection, and he had some large, fairly discrete cervical lymph glands, another strong indication for Tub. Bov., a dose of which was given in the 30th centesimal potency. There was no trouble examining on his next visit a month later, and his glands had substantially subsided. If Tub. Bov. is not otherwise indicated, the remedy may be one of many. It saves time to eliminate; Tub. Bov. first.

Fastidiousness
Most children are untidy, some extremely so, in which case, especially if the child can never keep clean for any length of time, Sulphur or Psorinum may be the constitutional remedy. If the child is extremely tidy, naturally putting his toys away in neat rows, this is a useful symptom

and the constitutional remedy is likely to be found among the following: Arsenicum, Anacardium, Nux. Vom., Graphites, or Carcinosin. Occasionally Phos., Sepia, or Platina may be indicated.

The value of being careful in assessing homoeopathic symptoms is illustrated by the following case. A child of four years used to smack his younger brother and this was attributed to jealousy. He was given Lachesis on this and other grounds, without benefit, and on careful questioning it was discovered that the older brother was fastidious and he smacked his brother's hands only when they were unclean. One of the fastidious remedies was prescribed with excellent results.

Fears

Very young children tend to fear noises more than anything else and babies start readily at sudden noises. If this symptom is to be taken it must be so marked that the baby 'almost jumps out of its skin'. Fear of the dark is common in childhood. The older the child, the more likely it is to be of value and if one child differs in this way from his siblings it gives more weight to the symptom as an individual one. As with any 'homoeopathic' symptom, it must be rejected as a repertorising symptom if there is any doubt of its value. To include doubtful symptoms is probably the most common error in inexperienced case-taking. Fear of downward motion may be manifested in babies by crying when lowered into the cot, and in older children from their reaction to going down in a lift. Fear of animals, of strangers, or of other children may be present. For children who cannot hold their own at school with other children, Silica, Carcinosin, Phosphorus or a Phosphorus compound will nearly always be found to cover the case, and if so, the fear almost invariably disappears.

Jealousy

This is within the average pattern of children, so that it must be assessed within their background.

Sensitivity to Reprimand

Dr Twentyman pointed out that the mental characteristic of the sycotic group of remedies was 'shame', and of the syphilitic group 'fear'. For some years now I have used 'sensitivity to reprimand', i.e. the child is terribly upset at being scolded even comparatively mildly, as a confirmatory symptom for Medorrhinum, Natrum Sulph. or any of the sycotic group, and can confirm the practical value of this observation.

Travel

Some children are much better when travelling in a car or bus or train, forgetting all about their troubles, even eczema. Nitric Acid is the chief remedy, or one of the others in the short rubric in Kent's *Repertory* under 'Riding in the car ameliorates'. Carsickness is worthy of note. While Cocculus 30c usually helps on a journey, the tendency can be used at least as a confirmatory symptom in constitutional prescribing.

In the section on Travel, under Mind, meaning desire to travel, it should be remembered that nearly all children like to travel, providing they do not get car sick. Only if there is almost a craving for travel can it be taken as an individual symptom.

The Family and Personal History

The two streams of heredity join at conception and from then on environmental influences begin to operate in utero. From the viewpoint of prescribing, the serial history is studied to find out if there is anything outstanding when regarded against a background of an 'average family and personal history'.

The Family History

A study of the antecedents of patients, mainly children, benefiting from Carcinosin strongly suggested that there was a greater tendency to cancer, tuberculosis, diabetes, or a combination of these, than average. This knowledge can be utilised in prescribing. In the case of a child suffering from recurrent attacks of high fever after tonsils and adenoids had been removed, and all investigations were negative, a history of diabetes on both sides of the family suggested Carcinosin, and this was confirmed by the child's appearance and other symptoms. Carcinosin 30c, one dose, was given over a year ago and there has been no recurrence of the fever. From a practical point of view, this knowledge of Carcinosin was of more value to me than anything else regarding the family history. There must surely be much more to be learned.

Pregnancy

It is not very often that one can get help from the history of pregnancy or labour, although the period of gestation and birth must be of great importance. The following factors merit consideration:

Infection. Influenza and other infections can cause abortion. German measles certainly and probably other infections may result in congenital abnormalities. It is reasonable to assume that infection of the mother could influence the foetus less drastically, yet leave its mark, just as post-natal infections are capable of leaving an aftermath of ill-health.

Trauma. Physical trauma may directly affect the foetus, and possibly also severe emotional disturbance of the mother.

Drugs and X-rays. The mother may be given iron, some preparations of which may be toxic, antibiotics, steroids, hormones, prophylactic immunisation, and occasionally anaesthetics for an operation. The mother may smoke heavily or be addicted to alcohol. Whether we can make practical use of the history in this respect is doubtful at present. A history of drugs should certainly be taken. The central nervous system depressant drugs generally seem to have the effect of blocking thinking in sensitive subjects. X-rays are now strongly suspect. Neither X-ray or Radium Bromide in potency has had any effect in stopping the inevitable downward course of leukaemia in my experience; but in less serious conditions, X-ray 30c or 200c may help if the case is hanging fire in spite of careful prescribing, and if there is a history of exposure.

Endocrine disturbance. It is well known that diabetes mellitus can influence the foetus and it is likely that other endocrine dysfunctions such as hyperthroidism may also do so.

In asking about pregnancy, therefore, it may be worthwhile to enquire about any acute illness, drugs taken, the habits of the mother with regard to smoking and alcohol, exposure to radiation, physical trauma, emotional upsets, operations and anaesthetics.

Labour
The infant may be subjected to drugs, including anaesthetics, and physical injury. If there is a history of slow or precipitate labour, the use of forceps, and/or slowness in recovery from birth, or difficulty in taking solids later, the head injury remedies – Natrum Sulph., Natrum Mur. or Cicuta – may be required. Unfortunately the effects of cerebral anorexia are irreversible. The mother is often in a highly suggestible state during labour, and whether suggestion at this time can influence the infant or not is unknown.

Post-natal History
A record is made of any outstanding event in the medical history since birth, including undue reaction to prophylactic immunisation, severe infections, injury including operations, frights or other emotional disturbances, effects of drugs and anaesthetics, general or local, and whether or not the episode immediately preceded ill-health.

When there is a history of severe reaction to vaccination, or ill-health appears to date from it, especially when symptomatically indicated remedies fail to benefit properly, Thuja may be considered as a pathological remedy. In any case in which there is a very large scar it is useful to make a note of it, as it might be useful as a confirmatory symptom. A bad reaction to vaccination is possibly of less value in an allergic subject than in others.

Thuja does not bear the same relationship to other inoculations. Sometimes a potency of the appropriate vaccine helps, but it may fail completely. There is need for study here.

When there is a history of a severe attack of one of the childish illnesses, such as measles or whooping cough, it may be necessary to antidote this by the appropriate nosode. The nosodes Morbillinum, Pertussin, Scarlatinum, Diphtherinum, Parotidinum, etc. may be dramatically effective or else have no effect. There is a generally accepted principle of homoeopathic prescribing that the remedy which was indicated at the time of an acute illness, but not given, can be effective years later in clearing up an aftermath of ill-health. An outstanding example of this is Drosera, a pathological remedy for whooping cough, and it is probably more useful than Pertussin in this respect. It is usually impossible to find indications for the remedy which might have been required at the time of the acute episode.

Dr Tyler believed that Hahnemann's Psora probably consisted, not of the effects of a single specific infection, but represented the aftermath of one or more of any of the acute infections. Obviously, if this is true, these diseases and their antidotes deserve more attention than they are generally given in homoeopathic practice. Certainly Dr Tyler used these nosodes to great advantage, but often in patients who had received her skilled attention for some time previously. My impression is that the psychosomatically-chosen remedies should be tried first, and remedies whose selection depends on the serial history should be considered when the former fail to produce satisfactory results, except when there are no clear-cut indications for a single psychosomatic remedy. In such cases it is worthwhile to go back through the whole history, family history, the period of gestation, labour, and post-natal events as outlined, and consider the bowel nosodes. The after-effects of poliomyelitis, apart from irreversible pathological changes, may be helped by Lathyrus Sativa lM or an individual remedy. Glandular fever – either dragging on, or where there is a family history of glandular fever – calls for consideration of Carcinosin 30c, 200c or 1M, or all three on consecutive days. A few cases in which the ordinary remedies failed to help when whooping cough persisted for a long time also responded to Carcinosin.

When children have had an unusually large number of acute infections Carcinosin should again be considered.

B. Coli Mutabile 200c is a valuable remedy with which to clear up the end stages of urinary tract infection when there are no pathological barriers. It is possible that it might be useful in dealing with chronic pyelone-phritis, which is realised now to be not uncommon. For the more immediate after-effects of any acute infection, such remedies as Sulphur, Psorinum, Carbo Veg., etc. have to be taken into consideration before thinking of the nosode.

When a child's general health has been improved after an acute infection, Thyroidinum 200c usually helps later on, even in adult life, perhaps because there has been a good response to thyroxin liberated during the fever.

In dealing with the possible after-effects of a serious acute infection, it should be kept in mind that there may have been quite other disturbing factors operating simultaneously. For example, the child may have suffered more from grief, fright, or a sense of injustice at being taken into hospital or through a sadistic nanny. Possibly some of our failures are caused through lack of information on this aspect.

A history of fright may be antidoted by Opium CM. Sometimes it has to be surmised, as, for example, in cases of enuresis starting after being in hospital.

Causticum or Opium may help children who have been burnt. Again, Carcinosin is worthy of consideration in cases of severe fright, prolonged fear, or unhappiness.

Injury remedies may be required on the basis of the history.

It is worthwhile to enquire about drugs and anaesthetics, as occasio-nally, for example, when there is a history of difficult resuscitation from nitrous oxide, when Nitrous Oxide 200c may be tried.

Observation of the Patient

All experienced homoeopaths come to be able to recognise certain remedies in their patients almost at a glance, and quite often the choice of remedies may be narrowed down appreciably through some infor-mation obtained through the senses. For instance, obese children nearly always need Calc. Carb. or Graphites. A wrinkled forehead in childhood, especially in infancy, is almost always covered by one of the small group of remedies listed in Kent's *Repertory*. Innumerable examples could be given. The point I want to stress for the student is not to neglect this invaluable part of the case history. Some authors are particularly helpful. Dr Tyler's *Drug Pictures* contains much of value in this respect. Dr Elizabeth Wright Hubbard and Dr Margery Blackie have given us some excellent clinical remedy pictures. The best introduction is probably Dr Borland's *Children's Types*.

A SCHEME FOR PAEDIATRIC CASE-TAKING IN ACUTE DISEASE

A perfect scheme of case-taking has yet to be devised, but if the following headings are remembered, sufficient information can nearly always be obtained on which to base a prescription with or without the aid of a repertory.

Mode of Onset
This includes aetiological factors such as chill or fright. Also the rate at which symptoms develop.

Here it is appropriate to discuss 'pathological' remedies – remedies specially associated with aetiological factors or with pathological states. Examples are Arnica in the case of surgical shock, Ignatia in acute grief. The question is whether or not pathological remedies may be regarded as being in a separate category from individual remedies. If we take the above examples, it is a fact established beyond any reasonable doubt that Arnica and Ignatia are highly effective when given soon after the onset of symptoms. As time goes on, however, it may be necessary to give other remedies to some patients, remedies differing individually. When bruising persists an unduly long time, Sulphuric Acid may be required, and in other patients other remedies may be needed to aid full recovery from the effects of an injury. Similarly in the case of grief, Natrum Mur., Phosphoric Acid, etc. may be required later on an individual basis. It may be that pathological remedies cover the vast majority of immediate reactions to certain aetiological factors, and therefore they are still, strictly speaking, individual. If this concept is held, while it is extremely useful to have pathological remedies in mind, it is important to be on the look-out for any unusual response.

Mentals
This heading includes any marked mental symptoms which have appeared since the illness began, such as irritability, craving for affection, fear, etc., together with any outstanding mental characteristics

such as a dislike of consolation which has persisted into the acute illness. Delirium comes into this category, as well as dreams, if these are very vivid or repeated.

Physical Generals

Appearance of the patient, including decubitus, restlessness, fastidiousness, uncleanliness, the presence or absence of perspiration and if present, its distribution, the facial appearance, skin eruptions, etc.

Appetite – mainly in respect of thirst. Absence of thirst in fever is a high value symptom (chiefly Pulsatilla and Gelsemium). Thirst is normally present, and should be taken into consideration only if it is excessive or peculiar. A moderate desire for cold drinks is usual and of no prescribing value. Thirst for warm drinks is unusual and should be noted (chiefly Lycopodium or Arsenicum Album). Thirst for frequent sips of fluid is found chiefly in Arsenicum Album.

Reaction to heat and cold. Distribution of heat in the body.

Odours – of the skin, sweat, breath, urine, stools, discharges.

Modalities
Modalities pertaining to the patient are of much higher value than those pertaining to a particular, as a rule. Time modalities are important; also it is worth while to note any modalities related to the natural functions such as sleeping or eating.

Particulars (if outstanding)
While a scheme of case-taking is necessary, the best histories are nearly always obtained through careful attention to what the mother says, astute observation and little in the way of interrogation. What is wanted is not a mass of symptoms, but a picture of the individual reaction in proper focus with the few very definite symptoms in the foreground. One of the remedies which covers the few salient features will usually be found to cover all the rest. Finally, if there are little or no symptoms of reaction, Sulphur may be the remedy.

Chapter 8

The Management of Specific Conditions

Traumatic Conditions

Injury, including birth trauma, plays a significant part in disablement and death in infancy and childhood. Dr C. V. Pink, with thirty years' experience of obstetrics, considers that Arnica 30c or 200c given to mother and child after parturition, sometimes with Hypericum and in the same potency, is of service in helping both to overcome the effects of trauma. The effects of Arnica in preventing puerperal sepsis as well as overcoming the effect of injury is well known to homoeopaths who have used it for this purpose for generations. Gross cerebral haemorrhage kills, and minor shock requires no treatment, but there is a considerable margin of cases in between in which, to say the least, it is possible that the shock and after-effects of injury can be minimised. In head injury, if there are no specific indications for Natrum Sulph., Cicuta or Natrum Mur., it is worthwhile to consider Helleborus, the symptomatology of which is closely similar to the after-effects of head injury and which has clinically been found to be a near-specific.

Homoeopathy in the Children's Ward

Most children settle down quickly in the ward, but the very timid or tense or desperately homesick child can usually be given a homoeopathic remedy which will restore him to happiness. Phosphorus is the most commonly indicated remedy for the very frightened child. The Phosphorus child is responsive, loves affection and gives it out. Pulsatilla loves affection but is not so responsive. Calc. Phos. is another remedy with sometimes a craving for affection. Responsiveness, fear and hyperactivity of the senses are a triad of symptoms found in the Phosphorus child. The child often shrinks away when you go to examine her or asks, 'What are you going to do to me?' Phosphorus 200c or 10M is the routine prescription for pre-operative anxiety.

Sometimes Pulsatilla or Ignatia are required. The latter is occasionally invaluable when a very young child is separated from his parents and experiences acute grief because to him he has 'lost' his parents forever. The terribly tense child settles down on Dysentery Co. 200c. Capsicum 200c is the first remedy to think of in homesickness. Sometimes a child reacts to the new situation of being in the ward by developing dirty habits, and Sulphur 200c is almost always followed by a dramatic change for the better.

Acute Manifestations of Psychosomatic Disease
In the treatment of a child suffering from an attack of asthma, acidosis or other acute psychosomatic disorder, the approach is similar to the treatment of injury or acute infection – to observe the pattern of individual reaction and match this with a remedy, known from its provings and/or therapeutic record to be capable of dealing with it. In asthma, if no unusual pattern is followed, such as relief from lying down (Psorinum) or relief when kneeling in the knee-elbow position (Medorrhinum), Arsenicum Iodatum 6c six doses 1-hourly or 2-hourly is a useful routine prescription. In attacks of cyclical vomiting or other manifestation of the periodic syndrome, Dysentery Co. 30c or 200c six doses 2-hourly is useful in the mentally tense child who gets sick on excitement such as when preparing to go to a party, and for others Senna 6c six doses 2-hourly, as recommended by Dr Vannier of Paris. Phosphorus and Lycopodium are sometimes indicated in the attack. The treatment of these diseases is, however, essentially constitutional.

Pathology and Prognosis
In assessing the possible value of homoeopathy in any chronic condition a knowledge of the pathological state is of course required, although this in itself may not enable an accurate prognosis to be made. For instance, vitamin-resistant rickets can respond to homoeopathic treatment. That there is a constitutional factor in rickets is apparent because when the disease was common, one child in an institution might develop it and others in the same environment and having the same diet did not. Without change of diet or extra vitamin D, many of us have seen children suffering from rickets lose their night sweats and improve remarkably after a high potency of Calc. Carb., Phosphorus, Medorrhinum or other indicated remedy. The very fact that vitamin-resistant rickets exists is evidence that there is some other factor than the generally accepted pathology.

On the other hand, idiopathic epilepsy does not as a rule seem to be influenced by homoeopathy, although there may be no obvious pathological changes. To take another example, bronchiectasis is incurable, but constitutional treatment can raise resistance to infection to such an extent that the patient's outlook is appreciably improved – something of obvious value when the disease is widespread. Such a child who had lobectomy performed, but was too ill for further surgery, used to get pneumonia with every cold. Constitutional treatment (with Bacillinum mainly) was followed by a gain in weight of a stone in eighteen months and colds could be easily thrown off. We may fail in such cases, but homoeopathy has something of potential therapeutic value whenever raising of resistance is a problem.

Gestation

The period of gestation is regarded in homoeopathic practice as a time specially suitable for constitutional treatment of the mother. During pregnancy there may be an outcropping of constitutional symptoms not in evidence at other times. This includes craving for or aversion to articles of diet. Hahnemann recommended Sulphur to be given to the pregnant mother, to beneficially influence adverse heredity tendencies when there were no indications for anything else.

Infant Feeding

An infant's chance of survival is enhanced by breast-feeding. In premature infants the chance of survival is doubled in breast-fed as compared with the artificially-fed. Homoeopathy has a great deal to offer in conjunction with other measures such as pre-natal preparation by pulling out the nipples advocated by Waller to enable the infant to bite beyond the tender tip. The use of Calendula compresses for tender nipples; (a drachm of the tincture to a pint of water) sometimes enables breast-feeding to be maintained when sore nipples could be a cause for weaning. Phytolacca 6c or higher is valuable when there is pain radiating from the nipple and there are many other local and constitutional remedies to abort breast abscesses (such as Bryonia, Belladonna and Pyrogen), and other remedies to help effectively in maintaining lactation, including Pulsatilla, Calc. Carb., Zincum, Ignatia and many others. Here is a field for research, because if our clinical impressions are correct, homoeopathy could here also provide means for a major advance in paediatrics. In dealing with feeding mismanagement, having considered the diet and feeding technique, Carbo Veg. and Lycopodium are most commonly indicated when there is excessive flatulence or flatus.

Tonsils and Adenoids

A common problem in children is frequent colds, often associated with chronically infected tonsils and adenoids, or the latter with sinusitis and otitis media. Perhaps the main indications for operation are evidence of a septic focus which, especially when flared up, has a serious effect on the child's health, such as might be accompanied by loss of weight and/or persistent obstruction of the nose. In a great many cases the indication for operation may not be clear. Constitutional treatment is well worth while, even if operation is done later, as it raises the general level of health. It is seldom that dramatic results are obtained in such cases if there is a septic focus, but when, after operation, improvement is not apparent, constitutional treatment is usually successful, and the impression is that if such treatment has been given before operation the after-effects of surgery are better. There are many remedies which may be indicated in such cases. Kent advocated Tuberculinum for chronically-infected tonsils and adenoids; a strong indication for this remedy is very large tonsillar or other cervical glands, such as might make one think of tubercular cervical adenitis.

Constitutional Treatment of Psychosomatic Conditions

Purely spasmodic asthma responds relatively easily to treatment. (It is said that it should respond to psychotherapy alone.) When there is lung damage, progress is slower and sometimes incomplete. When there is also eczema, there may be even more difficulty, but in all conditions homoeopathy can play an effective part in treatment.

A wide range of remedies may be required. Medorrhinum is a remedy which is not infrequently indicated in asthma when the child has fewer or no attacks when at the seaside and adopts the knee-elbow position in an attack. Epilepsy and petit mal are sometimes classified as psychosomatic disorders. These conditions do not respond as a rule well to homoeopathic treatment. The spasmodic remedies when indicated are worth special consideration. A case of petit mal in a child of eight, diagnosed at a children's hospital to be the result of encephalitis accompanying whooping cough, cleared up completely on Drosera 30c, 200c, 1M, but such is the exception rather than the rule.

Migraine responds well to constitutional treatment in adults, and even more readily in children. It is not very common before puberty. Cyclical vomiting and other manifestations of the periodic syndrome which can be regarded as the equivalent of migraine respond well to homoeopathic treatment, both in an attack and in preventing recurrences. Commonly-

71

indicated constitutional remedies are Phosphorus, Tuberculinum, Calc. Phos., Carcinosin and Dysentery Co.

Enuresis calls for a careful examination and a full investigation of psychological and environmental factors. The over-stern father or the big brother reading at night, keeping the small brother awake until he falls into too deep a sleep, for example, must be dealt with. In addition to all other measures, homoeopathy can play a very definite part in treatment, which should be constitutional; local application of Hypericum ointment or lotion, if there is rawness, is sometimes also useful. When Tuberculinum is indicated, Bacillinum Testium is reputed to be the best preparation. When all other measures have been exhausted, as is sometimes the case, Polyvalent Bowel Vaccine may help. The effect of treatment in a condition which tends to cure itself is difficult to assess.

Chronic Indigestion
Chronic indigestion in one form or another takes up a considerable amount of the paediatrician's time. Constitutional treatment can play a very useful part in this condition. There are the already-mentioned adverse effects of aluminium cooking utensils in undermining the health of a minority of children. This has special importance in alimentary disorders and allergic diseases. Common symptoms are irritability, touchiness about the least thing, slowness in eating, accompanied by a sensation as if food lodged behind the sternum, and itching of the eyes, especially the inner canthi. A specially important feature of aluminium is weakness of the rectal muscles so that straining is necessary for the evacuation of a stool of normal consistency. Dryness of mucous membranes and skin along with a tendency to cracking of the skin may also be present.

A girl of eleven years of age came to the hospital with the complaint of diarrhoea, alternating with constipation since the age of eighteen months. She had almost constant headaches and a leucorrhoeal discharge for six years. All the aluminium symptoms mentioned were present. The cooking utensils were replaced by enamelware and the girl given a 200th potency of Alumina. Within a month all symptoms, including the leucorrhoea had disappeared and the irritable disposition vanished also. Incidentally, many migraine sufferers are extremely sensitive to aluminium, and it is advisable to make sure that the kettle is replaced as well as the pans.

Cyclical Vomiting

It has been estimated that 30 per cent of all children attending outpatients suffer from the group of conditions known as periodic vomiting, cyclical vomiting or bilious attacks. The average age of onset is three to seven years and there is a tendency to spontaneous cure at puberty. Some writers recognise a periodic syndrome which may manifest itself as periodic vomiting or headache, or abdominal pain, or fever, or diarrhoea with pale stools.

. The classical type of cyclical vomiting occurs at very regular intervals, and is accompanied by severe ketosis. Irregular attacks may be included under this heading, as well as recurrent attacks of ketosis associated with upper respiratory infection. There are two main clinical types with many variations and combinations. First, there is the child who has regular or irregular attacks every few weeks or at longer intervals of feeling off colour for a day or two, followed by vomiting, upper abdominal pain, headache, furred tongue and constipation. The breath and urine smell strongly of acetone. There is a temperature of 38.5°C or so, occasionally it goes up to 40.5°C. Tonsillitis is often present. The condition passes off after two or three days. The other type is the highly-strung nervous child, often an only child, thin, stooping, intelligent, but lacking in concentration. He also has vasomotor instability and becomes suddenly pale. He gets an attack on excitement such as anticipation of going to a party. Eggs and cream given as extra nourishment aggravate matters. Cream is a special offender, and such children should be given skimmed milk. Cyclical vomiting is not infrequently met with in families with a history of migraine. In some cases at puberty, instead of clearing up, the attacks of acidosis merge into attacks of migraine.

The homoeopathic treatment of this and allied conditions resolves itself into two parts; treatment during the attacks, which is the less important, and constitutional treatment in between attacks to alter the patient so that he does not tend to have them. During an attack a number of remedies including Phosphorus, Pulsatilla and Dysentery Co. may be indicated. Constitutional treatment embraces a wide range of remedies and is highly effective in reducing the number and severity of attacks, and in most cases eventually wiping them out altogether. Phosphorus, Calc. Phos., Tuberculinum and Dysentery Co. have been frequently indicated in such children, but the treatment depends, as all constitutional treatment does, on the individual patient's mental and physical make-up. In one case, the child was so prone to car sickness that the mother stated he could not ride in a bus or car for more than ten minutes without being violently sick. There were other constitutional indications for Cocculus and it was given as a preliminary medicine. Not only did the car sickness clear up, but the cyclical vomiting did too.

There is one remedy, however, which is invaluable in many cases of cyclical vomiting, and that is Dysentery Co. My attention was drawn to it by a boy who had pyloric stenosis for which Ramstedt's operation had been performed with success, but he later developed cyclical vomiting which was rapidly cured by giving Dysentery Co. as a constitutional remedy. I found Dysentery Co. 30c to CM, usually the 200th potency, so useful both in attacks and between attacks that I almost came to regard it as a specific. 'Nervous tension', which Dr Paterson stresses as the charateristic mental state of Dysentery Co., is frequently found among these highly-strung children who get an attack on excitement. I usually prescribe the remedy 200c three doses two-hourly, followed by three doses four-hourly at the commencement of an attack.

This use of Dysentery Co. was, I found, no new discovery. In an old paper by Dishington it is noted as having a clinical record in recurrent bilious vomiting. The use of Dysentery Co. in abolishing, so to speak, over-action of the sympathetic part of the automatic nervous system led to its use in a much rarer kind of recurrent vomiting. A girl of four years was seen in the outpatients' department, sent up because she had been having attacks of pain in the left side of the abdomen followed by vomiting nearly every weekend for the previous six months. There was abundance of acetone in the breath and urine during these attacks. Pain of a severe nature preceding vomiting and in the left side of the abdomen strongly suggested that this was not simply a case of cyclical vomiting. During the two or three days while the pain was severe, there was an oliguria and polyuria ensued as the attacks passed off. Examination revealed an enlarged left kidney, and an intravenous pyelogram showed dilation of the calyces. Dysentery Co. 200c given two-hourly at the commencement of an attack aborted it, and after a few attacks were aborted in the same way they stopped altogether. This child has had no attacks for over two years. She is now seven. Blood pressure readings were made periodically in case a hypertension might develop, but the pressure has remained normal. The left kidney is now no longer palpable and the child seems very well.

Feeding Mismanagement
Because of the excellent work done in health centres, problems of feeding mismanagement are now relatively few in hospital practice, but

they do occasionally arise. A breast-fed baby of three months was admitted to Barton Ward suffering from diarrhoea and vomiting. It is rare indeed to have non-specific diarrhoea (the old summer diarrhoea) in breast-fed babies. Out of a series of over 200 cases admitted to Great Ormond Street Hospital, only one was breast-fed. Breast-feeding was continued while the infant was in the ward. No pathogenic organisms were found in the stools. Test weighing showed that the baby was receiving the proper amount of breast milk, but on observing the technique of feeding it was discovered that the mother was not bringing up the wind properly. No other treatment was given than to demonstrate the right way to do this. The baby was discharged within four days and there has been no further trouble.

A bottle-fed infant of four months brought to the outpatients' department with the complaint that he had been vomiting after nearly every feed for two months and had offensive diarrhoea and sleeplessness for one month. The technique of feeding was checked and it was readily ascertained by tipping up the feeding bottle that the hole in the teat was far too small. Secondly, the young mother was not expert at bringing up wind. The infant's expected weight and actual weight coincided. He was being fed with a correctly balanced milk mixture but was getting 48 oz. in the day instead of 34 oz. In other words, he was being considerably overfed.

The strain of mismanagement was beginning to tell. The hole in the teat was altered and the mother was shown how to bring up wind. The feed was reduced to 34 oz. He was given Lycopodium 30c, t.d. 3 days, b.d. 4 days, on the following grounds: wrinkled forehead; aggravation in the evening; objection to any feeds which were the least bit cool and a tendency to sweat about the face. There was also excessive flatus but this might not be a high-ranking symptom under the circumstances. Finally, his grandfather, who was an old outpatient of mine, was a typical Lycopodium subject. Occasionally useful clues may be obtained in selecting a young child's remedy by finding out which member of the family the infant takes after, and then taking their constitutional remedy into consideration. This baby gained twelve ounces during the next week and diarrhoea, vomiting and insomnia disappeared.

The use of Carbo Veg., Lycopodium and other remedies may be invaluable, but whatever homoeopathic treatment is given the diet and technique of feeding must be put right. On the other hand there are cases when nothing but constitutional treatment will enable the infant to digest his food.

Disorders of Personality

Stammering is, in my experience, difficult to treat by homoeopathy. Tics, anxiety states and the nervous child usually respond well. Silica is the most commonly indicated remedy for children who cannot hold their own with the other children, Phosphorus probably comes next. The excessively obstinate child, the kind of child Dr Tyler used to call the 'NO' child, usually responds to Tub. Bov.

Mental Handicap

It is very worthwhile to consider homoeopathic treatment in the case of the mentally handicapped child. Obviously the prognosis ultimately depends on the pathology. Down's syndrome cannot be altered basically, but constitutional treatment, except in a minority who presumably have a primitive brain formation, enables the individual to accept an education. Nearly all benefit definitely, physically and mentally, by receiving constitutional homoeopathic treatment, and by this means the most can be made of the material available. Medorrhinum is a near specific; Carcinosin, Sepia, Baryta Carb. and other remedies may also be required.

Chapter 9

Homoeopathy in Paediatric Surgery

When homoeopathy is used as an adjunct to surgery, it is useful to have a planned pre- and post-operative routine but to depart from this as occasion demands. Advances in surgery, anaesthesia and pharmacology have combined to make operations safer, and for the child at least, less frightening. Generally speaking, the non-homoeopathic use of drugs is confined to their action on tissues, organs and secretions of the body or, in the case of chemotherapy, on micro-organisms. Homoeopathic treatment, on the other hand, can influence the patient as a whole, stimulating natural recovery and the raising of resistance against infection. It is thus of especial value in cases of debility, when there is prolonged sepsis or when a series of surgical procedures have to be carried out.

Arnica 30c is the routine pre-operative homoeopathic prescription because of its remarkable effect on shock. For pre-operative fear or anxiety, which is present in a small proportion of children, Phosphorus 200c is commonly indicated. It is a useful remedy in many acute conditions of childhood. As a rule one or other of two aspects of Phosphorus present themselves – 'fear', and what may be termed 'responsiveness'. Phosphorus is full of fears; of the dark, of being left alone, and it is a remedy to be considered for anticipation. Either the child comes into the ward frightened or has been in the ward some time and is obviously anticipating the operation. An older child may shrink away from the examining doctor, saying, 'What are you going to do to me?' The responsiveness manifests itself by a strong desire for affection similar to Pulsatilla, but Phosphorus gives out affection, too, whereas Pulsatilla simply absorbs it. The appearance of Phosphorus is nearly always characteristic, the bright eyes following every movement of the doctor or nurse, the child being acutely aware of all that is going on in the vicinity, sometimes even when seriously ill. Only rarely the picture is that of apathy. A desire for cold drinks may be present. Its absence does not contraindicate Phosphorus, but a definite desire for warm drinks is unusual. When this is present, such remedies as Arsenicum Alb. and Lycopodium may be required, but only occasionally.

Pulsatilla is probably the next most commonly indicated prescription for pre-operative anxiety in children. In very young children, when admission to the ward is equivalent to 'loss of loved ones', Ignatia may be very comforting. When a blanket of chemotherapy is the normal procedure, Pyrogen 200c pre- and post-operatively may hold good too; homoeopathic treatment may be effective when chemotherapy fails. Pyrogen may be invaluable in any condition in which there is a septic focus and toxaemia or septicaemia, whether after tooth extraction, in peritonitis, skin or urinary infection. Toxaemia plus a discrepancy between pulse and temperature is a very reliable guide to Pyrogen. Other symptoms may be present, such as restlessness, because the part lain on feels sore ('the bed feels hard'), or offensive odours.

An alternative to Pyrogen which appears to act very well in osteomyelitis or any condition in which there is a profuse discharge from a wound, is to take a bead of pus and place it in distilled water or alcohol and have it potentised to the 30th potency. It is then given in the same way as any other remedy, say t.d.s. for 3 days, followed by b.d. for 3 days. In some recent cases of osteomyelitis and otorrhoea with 'threatened mastoid' this treatment appears to be extremely helpful, in addition to chemotherapy. The use of vaccines for such conditions is a well-known method which has been to some extent neglected since the advent of chemotherapy. Dr Charles Wheeler believed that the indication for an autogenous potency was a profuse discharge.

Chemotherapy is valuable in dealing with overwhelming infection. Homoeopathy can be effective when there are insensitive pathogenic micro-organisms, and has none of the disadvantages of chemotherapy immediate or remote. Whenever chemotherapy is administered, homoeopathic treatment can also be given to raise resistance. It is thus of particular value in this respect in infancy and early childhood, as well as in cases of debility. There is no doubt that prolonged administration of crude drugs can lower vitality, but apart from the administration or presence of volatile oils, it seems that crude drugs do not directly interfere with the action of potentised remedies.

The removal of tonsils and adenoids is a common operation. In the Royal London Homoeopathic Hospital the tonsils are removed by dissection. The routine homoeopathic medication is Arnica 30c six doses four-hourly pre-operatively, and post-operatively Rhus Tox. 30c six doses four-hourly. Rhus Tox covers the kind of sore throat experienced after the operation, pain and stiffness worse on first movement, relieved by subsequent movement, together with the characteristic post-operative restlessness. Aspirin or nepenthe are not withheld if required, but are rarely needed. The homoeopathic treatment may be effective with adults, but is by no means so uniformly successful as it is with children.

The most common abdominal operation in childhood is appendicectomy. The same routine is followed – Arnica and Rhus Tox. For most orthopaedic operations or mastoidectomy, Arnica is given pre- and post-operatively.

Staphysagria is a remedy well known for its effects on patients who are unduly sensitive to the pain of a clean-cut wound. It is given routinely after circumcision. Very occasionally, Staphysagria is required when an abdominal or other operation wound is unduly painful for no obvious reason. A boy of eight years of age was unable to walk about because of pain in the wounds a week after a bilateral herniotomy had been performed. The mother happened to be in the hospital having the same operation, and on enquiring about the boy's disposition she said, 'He bottles things up'. Staphysagria 200c six doses four-hourly was given and next day he was running round the ward free from pain. For infected wounds, homoeopathy offers an alternative to chemotherapy. Such remedies as Hepar Sulph. or Silica may be indicated. Silica is well known for its value in discharging wounds – 'pus with a vent' – and may be indicated when there is a watery oozing from a wound. Sometimes there is little else to confirm the choice, but in children at any rate it is worth remembering that the feet of a Silica child are almost always sweaty.

The value of Calendula lotion or ointment in the healing of wounds is well known. For large wounds with loss of flesh, Calendula in the 30th or 200th potency administered by mouth is usually remarkably effective.

Constitutional prescribing may be required after operation for patients not recovering normally. Sulphur, Psorinum and Carbo Vegetabilis may be useful post-operatively, in the same way that these remedies may be required to aid recovery after acute illness when convalescence is slow. Sulphur is not infrequently indicated by a lack of prescribing symptoms and especially if the child is inclined to be unclean in its habits. Opium has the effects of fright when 'fear of the fright' remains; when the incident is recalled the patient becomes afraid. If a child has had enuresis or other psychosomatic illness beginning after discharge from a hospital it is worthwhile to remember Opium, if apparently indicated remedies fail. A girl of eight years of age was given crystalline penicillin 500,000 units six-hourly on account of a 'threatened mastoid'. After five days the temperature rose from 39.5°C to 40.5°C, yet there were no indications for operation. On enquiry it was discovered that the child was extremely frightened by the injections of penicillin. There were strong indications for Phosphorus, which was given in the CM potency, and penicillin was discontinued. Next day the temperature fell, and within three days the child was discharged from hospital.

Otitis media responds to such remedies as Hepar Sulph. 200c, which may be given on the usual indications, sensitive inflammations, better for warmth, and mental irritability, or in the absence of clear-cut indications for anything else. Pulsatilla, Chamomilla, Belladonna or Ferrum Phos. are sometimes required. Occasionally it is difficult to distinguish between Belladonna and Ferrum Phos. Among the differences are: (a) Belladonna has a full hard pulse, Ferrum Phos. has a soft, easily compressible pulse; (b) Ferrum Phos. tends to alternate flushing and pallor of the face; (c) the actual presence of pus strongly suggests Ferrum Phos. It was Dr C. M. Boger's 'specific' given in very high potency for otitis media. When the ear drum is bulging, paracentesis may be required. Such remedies as Capsicum or Silica may be helpful in relatively mild cases of mastoiditis, but when there are signs of severe toxaemia such as drowsiness, vomiting and a high W.B.C., operation is needed.

Chapter 10

Belladonna and Related Remedies in Diseases of Childhood

Belladonna

Belladonna is a fairly commonly indicated remedy for acute childish illnesses, much more so in the children's ward than Aconite, possibly because the Aconite stage may have passed before admission. This chapter attempts to give a brief bedside differential remedy diagnosis between Belladonna and other remedies which at times present a similar clinical picture.

The typical picture of Belladonna is that of a child with a high temperature, flushed face, throbbing carotids and with intense heat of the skin – 'heat remaining long after on the examiner's fingers' – a very strong confirmatory feature of Belladonna. There is often a considerable thirst for large quantities of fluid, occasionally a craving for lemonade or lemons. The mental state of Belladonna is, as a rule, that of blunted mental acuity, a dullness of the intellect accompanied by delirium. The patient is typically not afraid of anything in the environment but may be frightened by the characteristic violent delirium which is often present.

Aconite

Aconite may be prescribed on a history of chill or fright without waiting for the typical symptoms to appear. Colds coming on within a few hours of being chilled are nearly always covered by Aconite. Nux Vomica is another important remedy to be considered for colds following a chill, and is practically certain if the patient with such a history is intensely irritable and cannot keep warm. Occasionally Aconite presents a picture not unlike that of Belladonna, with red face, hot skin and dilated pupils, but as a rule the Aconite pupils are contracted. Belladonna pupils are practically always dilated.

The Aconite mental state usually contrasts sharply with that of Belladonna. There is much less tendency to delirium in Aconite, and the patient is very alert and frightened, often of death. The Aconite patient may be extremely restless, whereas Belladonna may be intensely aggravated by movement. The anxiety and restlessness of Aconite may resemble that of Arsenicum, but there are usually clear distinctions in Arsenicum, such as a desire for warm drinks or frequent sips, periodicity, weakness out of proportion to the nature of the illness, and chilliness or fastidiousness.

Apis Mellifica

Apis Mellifica may present a red face, a very hot skin, indifference to surroundings, and delirium. Both have a tendency to start from sudden sharp pains. As a rule however Apis is much more alert mentally, and at first sight the appearance may closely resemble Phosphorus or a Phosphorus compound, the eyes following every movement in the vicinity. The Apis patient may want company too, but differs from Phosphorus in not being pleasant and in not wanting affection. The Apis patient is often miserable and whining.

An important difference which is nearly always present is that the face of Apis is of a rosy-red colour, rather than bright red. This rosy colour may be seen in the throat or on skin eruptions. This is very characteristic of Apis. Apis may be thirstless (sometimes after an initial misleading thirst), which may be accompanied by anuria. Together with a hot skin this triad is very suggestive of Apis.

A tendency to oedema is much more marked in Apis, as also is a late afternoon aggravation.

Baptisia

Baptisia resembles Belladonna in having a rapid onset, red face, hot skin and maybe delirium. The face of Baptisia, however, is a dusky 'besotted' red and mucous membranes are correspondingly darker.

Drowsiness and confusion are typical of Baptisia, and the patient may characteristically respond to questions, attempt to answer them but fall asleep before finishing. Occasionally the delirium of Baptisia gives a strong pointer, that of a sensation of being scattered about in the bed, or of having someone else in the bed. When this is present it is a useful confirmatory symptom.

Baptisia has the 'hard bed' sensation along with Arnica and Pyrogen. Sometimes, particularly in influenza, the distinction has to be made between Gelsemium and Baptisia. Gelsemium has a slower onset, a red face less often, heavy upper eyelids and sometimes thirstlessness. The mental state of Gelsemium typically is that of feeling 'miserable', in contrast to the dull confused mentality of Baptisia, although at times a differentiation may be difficult.

Bryonia

Bryonia may occasionally present itself with a red face and intensely hot skin. Both remedies have intense thirst, a dislike of movement and irritability, although irritability is much less often found in Belladonna. One difference is that Bryonia complaints are nearly always slower in developing. Whereas Aconite or Belladonna symptoms develop within hours, Bryonia symptoms commence a day or two after exposure, say, to a chill, and may take another day or two to fully develop.

The delirium of Belladonna is typically more violent, crowds of images pour in of animals, monsters, faces, etc. The delirium of Bryonia has been described as 'muttery delirium' and it does not usually disturb the patient very much. Delirium or dreams of work or of school in a child, or of being away from home, are characteristic of Bryonia.

Ferrum Phosphoricum

Ferrum Phos. may present a very similar picture to Belladonna, including intense heat of the skin, but differs chiefly in that Ferrum Phos. has the mental alertness of Phosphorus and responsiveness to every environmental influence, in marked contrast to the lack of interest in the environment of Belladonna. The face of Ferrum Phos. tends to flush up, alternating with pallor. Circumscribed redness of the cheeks is found in Ferrum Phos., the face of Belladonna is uniformly red, except sometimes there is a circumoral pallor.

The pulse of Belladonna is full and bounding, that of Ferrum Phos. is nearly always soft. Finally, if there is still a doubt, it is worthwhile to remember that Ferrum Phos. covers a later pathological stage, as for example in otitis media, when pus has definitely formed.

Lycopodium

Lycopodium likewise may resemble Belladonna, but the following points usually serve to differentiate. Firstly, Lycopodium may have a wrinkled forehead, a strong pointer to one of the remedies listed under this heading in Kent's *Repertory* – in childhood especially. Among these, Lycopodium is perhaps the most often indicated in acute illness. Secondly, the 4-8 p.m. aggravation is quite often present. Thirdly, Lycopodium nearly always has flatulence in acute disease of children. There is often some abdominal distention and eructation or frequent passing of flatus, usually the latter. Lycopodium is characteristically a right-sided remedy and is prominent among remedies covering symptoms going from right to left. If the generals are covered, however, it acts equally well in left-sided complaints, as for example in pneumonia.

Lycopodium may want cold drinks, but if a desire for warm drinks is expressed, Lycopodium or Arsenicum Alb. are the most likely remedies.

Nux Vomica
Nux Vomica occasionally resembles Belladonna in having a very red face and intensely hot skin. Other features of Nux Vomica may be present, but when there is a close resemblance, the most valuable differentiating point is that Nux Vomica cannot bear to be uncovered, despite the intense heat.

Opium also may resemble Belladonna, but differs in having pin-point pupils and often a blowing out of the lips on expiration when there is a high temperature.

Pulsatilla
Pulsatilla may have a red face, intense heat of the skin and sometimes considerable delirium, although delirium is not nearly so common as in Belladonna. The choice of Pulsatilla can nearly always be made on the mentals and generals. Typically the Pulsatilla child is weepy, has changeable moods, is sometimes touchy, but never violently irritable, and the main mental symptom in children – a desire for affection – is usually marked. In contrast to Phosphorus or a Phosphorus compound, the Pulsatilla child absorbs affection but does not give it out. Thirstlessness during fever is found in a number of remedies, but Pulsatilla and Gelsemium are certainly among the chief ones in childhood.

Pyrogen
Pyrogen does not often resemble Belladonna but it can have a red face and an intensely hot skin. Pyrogen usually differs from Belladonna in being more mentally alert and there is less delirium. In fact, Pyrogen has more often to be differentiated from the Phosphorus group. Sometimes in severe infections such as peritonitis or osteomyelitis the distinction may be virtually impossible. Fortunately the two are complementary and may be prescribed alternately, a justifiable procedure in such circumstances. Other differences betwen Pyrogen and Belladonna are that Pyrogen may be very restless and have offensive odours, features rarely found in Belladonna.

Stramonium
Stramonium may have a red face, dilated pupils, high fever, intense heat of the skin and delirium. Some cases may be difficult to distinguish from Belladonna, but as a rule this is not so. Generally, Stramonium has more

motor activity, while both cover jerking of limbs and convulsions; this tendency is much greater in Stramonium. Graceful movements of limbs, sometimes a guide in chorea, are found in Stramonium. The Stramonium child raises his head frequently from the pillow, whereas Belladonna nearly always keeps still and may be intensely aggravated by movement.

There is a greater tendency to loquacity in Stramonium, as great as in Lachesis. As Boericke puts it, 'Devout, earnest, ceaseless, talking. Loquacity, garrulousness, laughing, singing, sweating, praying, rhyming.' are features of Stramonium. There may be rapid changes of mood from joy to sadness. Lewd talk or religious mania are covered by both, but much more often by Stramonium. Grasping of the genitalia is not recorded under Belladonna.

In keeping with greater motor activity, the delirium of Stramonium may be as violent or even more violent than that of Belladonna, and its content may sometimes help in differentiating. There may be delusions of personal identity, of being tall, or being in two parts, or of a part of the body being enlarged or missing. (Baptisia, Petroleum and Phosphorus have delusions of the body being scattered about the bed.) Belladonna on the other hand typically sees faces, monsters, etc.

The face of Stramonium is sometimes pale with wrinkled forehead, but when it does resemble Belladonna, there may be contracted pupils, very rarely found in Belladonna. Circumscribed redness of the cheeks is not found in Belladonna. A frightened expression is prominent under Stramonium but not in Belladonna. Both have fear of water but this is more marked in Stramonium, which has also fear of running water. Stramonium has marked fear of the dark, not prominent in Belladonna, which is typically indifferent to surroundings. Violent pain in the left hip is occasionally a pointer to Stramonium.

A differential diagnosis may have to be made between Belladonna, Stramonium and Hyoscyamus. As a rule the temperature is lower in Hyoscyamus, but a detailed comparison will be necessary.

Sulphur

Sulphur may give an initial impression of Belladonna, with red face, hot skin and delirium, but on closer assessment of such cases it is realised that the characteristics of Belladonna are lacking. The pupils may be normal in size, probably more often than they are dilated or contracted. The heat of the skin may not be so marked as the intense heat of Belladonna. On a more careful look, it is realised that there is little or nothing in the way of prescribing symptoms. 'Absence of symptoms' is a well-known feature of Sulphur. There is just a patient plus the disease, be it measles or pneumonia, without any apparent manifestation of reaction except fever. This is a very valuable pointer to Sulphur at any stage of an acute illness, at the beginning or towards the end, when the storm has passed and the patient is not quite well, but there is a paucity or absence of prescribing symptoms.

Psorinum has been depicted as a chilly Sulphur, but the resemblance may be so close that Psorinum may be given successfully when Sulphur seems to be indicated but fails. Several remedies have 'despair of recovery', but in convalescence Psorinum is the only recorded one. It would seem that the sluggishness of the tissues is reflected in the mind. The Tuberculins also may closely resemble Sulphur. When a patient is slow in recovering from a pneumonia without any definite prescribing symptoms, Bacillinum seems to work very well.

To return to differences between Sulphur and Belladonna, Sulphur may have circumscribed redness of the face, a symptom not found in Belladonna. Recurrent flushing of the face is found in Sulphur. Very red lips are found in Sulphur and Tuberculinum. Sulphur also has extreme redness of other orifices. Sometimes the Sulphur patient has extreme heat of the feet, having to uncover them, a symptom not found in Belladonna.

One of the most common pointers to Sulphur is untidiness and uncleanliness. This is so strongly marked in Sulphur that when a child seems to take a delight in being dirty, Sulphur can almost be guaranteed to rectify this.

Veratrum Viride

Veratrum Viride may have a rapid onset of fever, red face, hot dry skin, dilated pupils and great thirst, together with frightening delirium. As Borland pointed out, Veratrum Viride tends to be cyanosed and to have a slight sweat on the face.

Slight nausea is often present. Borland also noted that some patients who responded to Veratrum Viride complained of 'everything tasting sweet'. The tongue may provide a pointer. A red tongue with a stripe of fur down the centre is typical of Veratrum. It is possible to have this in Belladonna, but very rarely. A dirty yellow tongue also suggests Veratrum. Belladonna usually has a clean tongue, not infrequently a 'strawberry' tongue.

Chapter 11

Phosphorus in Acute Diseases of Infancy and Childhood

The appearance of the Phosphorus child is usually helpful. The child is tall and slim with fine skin, and this is a guide in acute as well as in chronic conditions. A characteristic symptom is the way the child follows with his eyes every movement of the doctor or nurse, even when suffering from considerable toxaemia. Indifference or apathy is not common. This acute awareness of the surroundings is one of the most reliable symptoms and is rarely absent. Less often, hyperacuity of the senses is apparent by emphasis on sensitivity to noise or touch. The position in bed adopted by the Phosphorus patient is relatively unimportant – except for two positions. It is useful to remember that Phosphorus has the knee-elbow position along with some other remedies. Also, in pneumonia or other chest conditions the child may have a marked preference for being well propped up, sitting almost upright with the head thrown back.

Linked up with awareness is what might be called responsiveness, it is well known that the Pulsatilla child often craves affection; Phosphorus very frequently has this too, but with a difference usually easy to detect. The Pulsatilla child absorbs affection, so to speak, but does not return it, whereas the Phosphorus child responds by giving out affection. Phosphorus returns affection. The Phosphorus child is responsive to every external stimulus.

Silica and Phosphorus may have to be distinguished. Both have fear and just occasionally, like its relative Pulsatilla, Silica may crave affection. There are many differences, including the tendency to a sickly pale face in Silica and persistent discharges. Offensive sweat of the feet, often cold, or at least cold clammy toes, is a useful confirmatory symptom of Silica. Its absence would make one query the prescription.

Also linked up with the acute awareness of Phosphorus is apprehension or fear. Phosphorus is said to be full of fears – fear of the dark, fear of being left alone, of what the doctor is going to do, are common symptoms. It is almost always the correct remedy for pre-operative anticipation in children, including a visit to the dentist. It is so often indicated that it is given routinely for this condition unless there are positive indications for another remedy. About one in twelve children undergoing tonsillectomy require it. I give Phosphorus 200c, a single dose if time does noťpermit more, but usually a few doses are given two-hourly. It seems to work perfectly well along with the routine Arnica 30c. Phosphorus is one of the homesick remedies when the general symptoms agree.

The main symptoms suggesting Phosphorus in my experience are the four just mentioned – the appearance of the child, the eyes following every movement in the vicinity, responsiveness, and maybe fear. There is almost always some degree of fear or anticipation more prominent in some than in others. In a minority it is the main presenting symptom. Once the Phosphorus picture is really recognised, not just the adding up of symptoms, it is, as in other remedies, the most helpful guide to its prescription.

Usually there are other confirmatory symptoms such as desire for cold milk. Phosphorus is often thirsty for cold drinks in large quantities. A desire for warm drinks is a symptom which should make one hesitant in prescribing it. In such cases the most likely remedies are Arsenicum Alb., Lycopodium, or one of the others having a desire for warm drinks. Sometimes one can be misled by the mother giving a history of a desire for warm drinks when in fact she has given only warm drinks, supposing that cold drinks might be harmful. A desire for cold milk is a good symptom of Phosphorus, but a desire for cold drinks is usual in children suffering from fever and therefore is not a high value symptom. A desire for frequent sips of liquid is a strong pointer to Arsenicum Alb., but occasionally other remedies including Phosphorus may be indicated. Thirst for cold drinks which are vomited about ten minutes later is a well-known pointer to Phosphorus or Pyrogen. The combination of intense thirst and aversion to touch may suggest Bryonia, but the appearance and mental symptoms are very different.

The impression of constriction of the chest out of proportion to physical signs is often present in pneumonia, bronchitis and asthma when Phosphorus is indicated. The tendency to bleed is also a well-known feature of the remedy; it seems to be useful after tonsillectomy when there is oozing of bright red blood not sufficient to require ligation.

The toxic effects of Phosphorus on the liver are well known and the remedy covers the majority of cases of infective hepatitis in children.

Calc. Phos. and Ferrum Phos. are by far the most likely of the Phosphorus compounds to give an initial impression of Phosphorus.

They may both have the alertness – 'eyes following the doctor', responsiveness, and perhaps fear. 'Consolation aggravates' is very much less common. Almost always, however, the Calc. Phos. child is of heavier build and tends to have localised perspiration, usually on the head. Phosphorus may have localised perspiration, but more often has a mild, generalised, slightly sticky faint sweat, if sweat is present. The Calc. Phos. patient tends to have trouble, especially during dentition, and bronchitis during dentition is very often covered by Calc. Phos. Pneumonia apparently related to primary dentition does not occur very often, but for any complaint it is a remedy to be considered during dentition.

Ferrum Phos. may closely resemble Phosphorus in some cases, the only difference being a marked tendency to easy flushing of the face, or the patient presents a picture making one think of Phosphorus and Belladonna. Not infrequently the appearance, alertness, etc., of Phosphorus is present together with the intense heat of the skin so strongly suggestive of Belladonna – heat remaining long after on the examiner's fingers. Circumscribed redness of cheeks or alternating pallor and flushing of the face may be present in the Ferrum Phos. patient.

Sometimes Belladonna-like symptoms predominate, and in fact it may be difficult to decide on the remedy. The full bounding pulse of Belladonna is absent in Ferrum Phos. Ferrum Phos. is more useful at a later pathological stage, as for example when pus has definitely formed in otitis media. Ferrum Phos. may want warm drinks – a symptom rarely if ever found in Phosphorus. Ferrum Phos. was indicated in two cases of follicular tonsillitis. Both children had the Phosphorus appearance and mentals, together with circumscribed redness of cheeks plus intense heat of the skin. Both had a temperature of 40°C, and with that degree of fever the children would almost certainly have been dull mentally and delirious if Belladonna were the remedy. One of the children was a boy of 8 years of age, the son of a doctor friend who described the effects of Ferrum Phos. 200c as 'miraculous'. The other was a boy, 12 years old, who was admitted to Barton Ward with follicular tonsillitis and mesenteric adenitis, and there was evidence from the history and radiologically of a resolving bronchopneumonia. He had a white blood count of 38,000. Ferrum Phos. 10M was followed overnight by a considerable improvement. Pyrogen 200c completed the treatment and within three days his throat was free from Vincent's organism and his temperature and pulse had returned to normal.

Among the remedies occasionally to be distinguished from Phosphorus are Arsenicum Alb. when fear predominates, although other symptoms such as desire for warm drinks, restlessness and periodicity will usually make the decision fairly easy. Kali Phos. may very rarely be similar, but symptoms from the Kali element, such as 3 a.m. aggravation, intense reaction to noise, will be apparent sooner or later. Psorinum may have a Phosphorus-like appearance as well as the unwashed look. Dysentery Co. may simulate Phosphorus, and only after observation in the ward does it become apparent that mental tension is the keynote.

Zincum may give a strong initial impression of Phosphorus, but the history and restless feet or other characteristic symptoms of Zincum usually make the distinction easy. The Tuberculinums may also resemble Phosphorus, but intense obstinacy – which in a child almost always calls for Tub. Bov. – or other symptoms usually make the selection straight-forward. Tuberculinum follows Phosphorus as a complementary remedy.

Finally, it would seem that Pyrogen and autogenous pus potencies are frequently indicated in patients of the Phosphorus type, and I have not hesitated to alternate these remedies with apparent success.

Chapter 12

Carcinosin: A Clinical Proving

It is generally accepted that we can utilise the symptoms derived from clinical experience of the therapeutic effects of a remedy, and that the remedy picture which is the real basis of prescribing is built up from provings plus clinical experience.

My interest in Carcinosin was aroused by a chance experience in 1952, that of having in the outpatients' department simultaneously two children, a boy and a girl born of mothers who were, during pregnancy, suffering from cancer of the breast. The girl was the second child of first cousins with a strong family history of cancer. Both children presented a remarkably similar appearance, having blue sclerotics, café-au-lait complexion, and numerous moles – these were black, mostly circular macules, and any reference to moles in this book refers only to this type. I wondered if both these children exhibited these characteristics because of their mother's condition.

It would take a considerable time to collect a number of these cases, and the immediate course open was to study the antecedents of children either partially or completely of that appearance. In fact, comparatively few presented the full appearance, so children with moles, with or without the other characteristics, were included, and their family histories were compared with those of other children attending the outpatients' department and in the ward of the Royal Homoeopathic Hospital.

There was a higher incidence of cancer, tuberculosis and diabetes, or a combination of these, and to a lesser extent pernicious anaemia, in the family history of one hundred with moles, compared with a hundred children without moles; it would of course require more research to prove this.

After two hundred cases with apparently successful results of treatment with Carcinosin, the first paper, 'A Clinical Study of Carcinosin', was read to the Faculty of Homoeopathy. This led to a conventional proving by Dr Templeton, which elicited dullness of mind, thinking difficult, dissatisfaction (which was in keeping with Clarke's observation

91

that Carcinosin was useful in mental cases with a tendency to suicide), and a family history of cancer. The report of the proving was published in July 1958 along with the 'Carcinosin Drug Picture'. Dr Templeton deliberately took no part in the clinical proving, which however provided the indications for the use of Carcinosin in such cases, besides its main field of usefulness in the treatment of mentally normal patients.

After further study, the 'Carcinosin Drug Picture' paper was read to the Scottish branch of the Faculty in 1958, and the indications for Carcinosin have subsequently been abundantly confirmed. In the discussion on this paper, Dr Elizabeth Patterson said that she thought cancer represented the end effect of all miasms, which was why Tuberculinum, Medorrhinum and Lueticum were all needed. Dr Cooper said he thought of Carcinosin if there was a history of syphilitic heredity. He stated that he knew of a certain island which had an epidemic of syphilis in 1870, and that there was now much cancer, hypertension and mental illness of a depressive type.

Kent believed cancer to be a result of the suppressed psora, and it is of interest to note that in some cases responding to Carcinosin, clear-cut indications appear for a related remedy, including Psorinum.

I then studied the individual history of these children and found that there was a tendency to have an inflammatory illness, usually pneumonia or whooping cough, very early in life, say in the third month, and therefore almost always severely. If we accept McDonagh's concept that there are two basic diseases – inflammation and tumour formation – representing centrifugal and centripetal forces, and also the teaching of Rudolph Steiner, then one can regard this tendency to inflammation as a reaction against inherited tendencies.

A child with the longest list of severe infections I have ever seen had indications for Carcinosin, and its administration was followed by a remarkable improvement. Later on, Dr Imberechts, who had extensive experience, noted that a childish illness after puberty could be regarded as an indication for Carcinosin, and this I can fully confirm.

I lost touch with the 'original' girl but examined the 'boy' twenty-seven years later. He was generally fit and was following a professional career. It may be significant that he had developed DeMorgan's spots.

It soon became evident that after a prescription of Carcinosin there tended to be an inflammatory or other reaction, very often beginning on the tenth day, and that the reaction might last two or three weeks. This has been confirmed at all ages. It is better to assess progress six weeks after a prescription of Carcinosin rather than at four weeks, keeping in mind that if an aggravation should occur, it is virtually always completed by that time.

A pointer to the consideration of Carcinosin and other remedies in children may be found in the position that the child adopts in sleep. Up to about the end of the first year, sleeping in the knee/elbow position is not uncommon; after that it tends to decrease. If it persists, then it may be regarded as an individual symptom. This is important as it is unequivocal, as compared with parents' assessment of other symptoms, as to whether or not they are outside the norm. Enquiry in our outpatients' department, and observation in the ward, demonstrated that the following remedies cover this symptom: Calc. Phos., Carcinosin, Lycopodium, Phosphorus, Sepia and Tuberculinum, as well as Medorrhinum, which is the only remedy listed in Kent's *Repertory*.

Many of the patients being studied had already been receiving treatment, and it became apparent that candidates for Carcinosin in other respects had frequently been helped by one or more of a group of remedies, to which others have been added over the years. At the time of writing this list of related remedies is as follows:

Alumina	Natrum Mur.
Arsenicum Alb.	Natrum Sulph.
Arsenicum Iodatum	Nitric Acid
Bellis Perennis	Opium
Calc. Carb.	Psorinum
Calc. Phos.	Pulsatilla
Dysentery Co.	Sepia
Graphites	Staphysagria
Lachesis	Sulphur
Lueticum	Thuja
Lycopodium	the Tuberculinums
Medorrhinum	

In the case of a patient not responding to one of these remedies, although apparently accurately chosen, it is worthwhile to see whether Carcinosin may fit the case. Also, when two or more of the related remedies are strongly partially indicated, but no one adequately covers the case, Carcinosin should be considered.

Knowledge of related remedies is obviously very important. This cannot be summarised, but some outstanding mental or physical symptoms suggesting consideration of Carcinosin, together with reference to certain rubrics in Kent's *Repertory* to which Carcinosin can be added, are as follows:

Appearance. The full 'Carcinosin appearance' of blue sclerotics, café-au-lait complexion and black macules, already described, is rare. As in the clinical proving, the presence of these moles, with or without the other features, suggests consideration of Carcinosin.

Fear and Anxiety. One aspect of this is in children who cannot hold their own with other children at school. Such children can nearly always be cured by constitutional treatment, which in my experience mainly consists of Arsenicum Alb., Arsenicum Iod., Carcinosin, Phosphorus, Silica or Calc. Phos., according to individual indications. Sometimes more than one of these remedies are required. I usually prescribe these remedies in the 30th, 200th and 1M potencies, given on consecutive days. Fear and anxiety can of course be found in many other conditions and at all ages.

Anticipation. Dr Bon Hoa, who has extensive experience of Carcinosin, has not only confirmed this symptom, but in his valued opinion it is a very high-ranking one.

Desire for Affection. Remedies related to Carcinosin which may have a strong desire for affection are Pulsatilla, Phosphorus and Calc. Phos. The distinction is usually very obvious in children, in that the Pulsatilla child may absorb affection but does not strongly give it out. Phosphorus and Calc. Phos. usually return affection; Carcinosin covers either situation.

Sympathy to Others. In respect of a child, the mother can almost always tell. If in doubt about this symptom in an adult, it is sometimes useful to ask whether many people tend to ask their advice, or come to them when they are in trouble. At any age a close observer may settle the value of this symptom.

Deciding whether or not a symptom should be taken, as part of the basis on which a homoeopathic prescription is determined, is of the utmost importance. If there is any doubt regarding the value of any symptom it should be put aside. Really definite symptoms, however few, must be taken as a guide to the homoeopathic remedy; it is often difficult to make an assessment of this particular symptom. Kent's *Repertory* give the two rubrics 'Sympathetic' and 'Horrible things and sad stories affect her profoundly'.

Additions to the rubric 'Sympathetic' are as follows: Aurum Met., Carcinosin, Calc. Carb., Calc. Phos., Graphites, Helleborus Niger, Lachesis and Sepia.

Additions to the rubric 'Horrible things' etc. are Carcinosin and Nitric Acid.

Obstinacy. Tuberculinum is an important addition to this rubric, and Carcinosin can also be added. (Blue sclerotics has long been regarded as a symptom of Tuberculinum.)

Love of Travel. This is also covered by Carcinosin.

Sea Air. Rubrics covering amelioration or aggravation at the seaside are found in Generalities: 'Air, Sea'. Medorrhinum is the only remedy covering amelioration. Carcinosin can be added; both also cover aggravation at the seaside.

In the south of England a patient may find amelioration at the east coast and aggravation at the south coast, or vice versa; both situations are covered by Carcinosin.

In my experience, two remedies in the rubric 'Aggravation at the seaside' – Natrum Mur. and Sepia – can also cover amelioration. Silica, which is not listed, also can cover amelioration or aggravation.

Fastidious. Alumina, Anacardium, Bellis Perennis, Carcinosin, Conium, Graphites, Phosphorus, Platinum Met., Pulsatilla and Sepia. Arsenicum Alb. and Nux Vomica are also recorded in Kent's *Repertory.*

Sensitivity to Music. Carcinosin can be added to this rubric.

Enjoyment Watching a Thunderstorm. Kent records only Sepia in the rubric 'Sadness, thunderstorm ameliorates'. Bellis Perennis and Carcinosin can be added.

Sadness but Cannot Weep. This is covered by Gelsemium and Natrum Mur. Carcinosin can be added.

Dancing. See rubric of Mind, 'Dancing'. This means much more than the usual enjoyment, for example, dancing by oneself (apart from the tendency for young children to do so, unless very strongly marked). Carcinosin can be added to this rubric besides two remedies related to Carcinosin – Sepia and Lachesis.

Insomnia. The original children suffered from sleeplessness. Sometimes, and particularly when otherwise indicated, Carcinosin can be effective, but it does not prove an easy answer to this problem.

Foods. Craving or aversion to butter, eggs, fat meat, fat bacon, fruit, milk, salt and sweets is covered by Carcinosin. There may be a craving at one time and an aversion at another, or vice versa – not an uncommon finding in children. Obviously, in introducing new articles of diet there may be a temporary refusal, and this is within the norm. It is normal for most children to have a strong liking for sweets, and to take craving for sweets as a symptom it must be really definite. Aversion to sweets would be outside the norm in a child.

Symptoms Alternating from Side to Side. See Generalities, 'Side'. Carcinosin can be added to Lac Caninum and other remedies in this rubric. Other rubrics to which Carcinosin can be added are 'Cicatrices', 'Menopause', 'Vaccination', 'Wounds, Slow to Heal'.

Concussion After-effects. This is mainly covered by three rubrics in Kent's *Repertory* in the section on 'Head'.
1) Concussion.
2) Injury to the Head, After.
3) Pain Injuries, Mechanical, After.

A list of the remedies of these rubrics to which Alumina, Carcinosin, and Glonoin should be added can be used as a combined rubric in repertorising.

CARCINOSIN: A SUMMARY OF INDICATIONS FOR ITS CONSIDERATION

Appearance. Black macules, with or without blue sclerotics or café-au-lait complexion.

Family History. Judged to be outside the norm for incidence of cancer, leukaemia, tuberculosis and diabetes. Less frequently, pernicious anaemia, which is followed by a slightly higher incidence of cancer than average.

Past History. A childish illness such as whooping cough very early in life; and severe illness or a childish illness *after* puberty. Severe incident of prolonged whooping cough, glandular fever syndrome or vaccination, or prolonged after-effects. Post-menopausal illness.

Mentals and Generals. Fear and anxiety at any age, including children unable to hold their own at school. Anticipation may be a marked feature. Sympathetic to others, sometimes a craving for affection as well. Sensitive to music. Love of dancing. Sadness but cannot weep. (Carcinosin can be added to Gelsemium and Natrum Mur.) Enjoys watching a thunderstorm. See rubric 'Sadness, Thunder ameliorates'. Bellis Perennis and Carcinosin can be added to Sepia, which is the only one given in Kent's *Repertory* for 'Thunder ameliorates'.

Fastidiousness

Foods. Craving for or aversion to butter, eggs, fat meat, fat bacon, fruit, milk, salt, sweets. Sometimes there is a craving at one time and an aversion at another, which is not uncommon in childhood. Remember that in introducing new foods there is often an initial aversion.

Sea Air. Amelioration or aggravation.

Wounds Slow to Heal.

Scar Tissue.

Symptoms Alternating from One Side of the Body to the Other.

Related Remedies. Carcinosin should be considered if there is failure of a related remedy, although apparently well-indicated. Or when there are strong partial indications for two or more of the related remedies.

Post-Menopausal Illness.

Head Injury, After-Effect.

Chapter 13

The Carcinosins

Cancer nosodes have long been used before the clinical proving, mainly as constitutional remedies on the indication of a strong family history, and given with other remedies in the treatment of cancer. There is no record of a cure of cancer by a Carcinosin alone. The Carcinosin used in the clinical proving, unless otherwise stated, is said to have been derived from cancer of the breast. With the exception of Scirrhinum, I have pre-scribed Carcinosins derived from other sites in the treatment of disease occurring in the region of their origin, always provided that there were definite indications for Carcinosin.

My impression is that Carcinosins have a general common action, rather than the emphasis being on the location from which the specimen was obtained. Dr Twentyman considers that the level in the body from which the Carcinosin was obtained could be a guide to its local action. Experience has demonstrated that Carcinosin Adeno. Stom. has, for example, been highly successful in the treatment of many cases of chronic hepatitis, always when Carcinosin was otherwise indicated.

Carcinosin Adeno. Stom.
A man of eighteen presented himself for treatment on account of what had been diagnosed as sub-acute hepatic necrosis. Liver function tests indicated considerable liver damage; he was having frequent petechial haemorrhages and was being treated by a high protein diet only. After careful assessment I gave him Lycopodium 1M, four doses every twelve hours, but after three weeks it was obvious that little or no progress had been made. He then developed severe influenza and later on subcu-taneous abscesses, for which he was treated locally. Three months after the first consultation I saw him again and gave him Carcinosin Adeno. Stom. 30c, as careful assessment of the symptom complex still pointed to Lycopodium. This was followed by a great improvement. He began to get well, and after a year's careful treatment he began practising osteo-pathy, for which he had been training. Treatment was discontinued as it

did not seem necessary. Liver function tests reflected improvement, but did not come quite back to normal. Six years later he had an attack of glandular fever, from which he recovered after a course of Carcinosin Adeno. Stom. 30c t.i.d. for four days, then night and morning for three days. Obviously, in a disease known to be almost always self-limiting, his recovery might have occurred without treatment. (See also the chapter on 'Glandular Fever'.)

Car Sickness. Cocculus Indicus 30c is a near specific, one dose given just before the journey and repeated if sickness starts, and repeated, say, half-hourly for a few doses. Alternatively, tablets medicated with Staphysagria, Theridion, Petroleum, Cocculus and Tabacum 6c, two tablets to be taken at an interval of two hours before the journey, then at hourly intervals if required. This combination is sometimes also effective for sea sickness. In more severe cases constitutional treatment may be required, and given when not travelling, which should be avoided for a few weeks during which aggravation might occur. If travel is really necessary, the low potency mixture could be tried during that period. Should Carcinosin be constitutionally indicated, Carcinosin Adeno. Stom. 30c, three doses every six hours in one day, has been very effective in these cases.

Occasionally car sickness continues into adult life. A woman of fifty-six found it impossible to make a long car journey. There was a history of cancer of the throat on both sides of the family, and other symptoms pointed to Carcinosin. Carcinosin Adeno. Stom. 30c, three doses every six hours, was given to be taken in one day, and she was advised not to travel for a month. There was a considerable aggravation during the first week. There was no travel sickness for a few years when the prescription had to be repeated, again with excellent results.

Cyclical Vomiting A girl of five suffered from severe attacks of cyclical vomiting, previous treatment by paediatricians having failed. In this case both the father and the mother were diabetics, and the child had the full Carcinosin appearance – blue sclerotics, café-au-lait complexion and small black, mostly circular macules – plus other Carcinosin symptoms. Carcinosin Adeno. Stom. 30c was given, three doses every six hours in one day, and there were no more attacks.

Anxiety State When anxiety or anticipation – two prominent symptoms of Carcinosin – are felt in the epigastrium, Carcinosin Adeno. Stom. has been effective in a number of cases when Carcinosin was otherwise indicated.

Carcinosin Lung

In a few cases of recurrent bronchitis, Carcinosin lung has been extremely effective when indications for Carcinosin constitutionally were present. In the case of a woman of sixty-five, X-rays taken by the same radiologist on the same apparatus showed a definite diminution of scarring after treatment.

Carcinosin Breast

This nosode has sometimes been invaluable in chronic cystic mastitis. There was a recurrence in one of these cases some years later, which also responded well. In some cases Carcinosin was ineffective.

Carcinosin Bowel Co.

This was effective in many cases of rectal and anal conditions. Before the availability of Carcinosin Uterus, Carcinosin Bowel Co. was prescribed because of the site of its origin, with apparent success in a few cases of dysmenorrhoea to complement individual treatment given at the time of menstruation. (See also the chapter on Bellis Perennis.)

Scirrhinum

Described in Clark's *Dictionary* as a nosode of scirrhous cancer which was introduced by Dr Compton Burnett, who proved it on himself. It produced a tremendous sinking at the navel, which he regarded as a keynote for its use. He reported that Scirrhinum had aided in the cure of many cases of breast cancer. A patient to whom Burnett had given Scirrhinum mentioned that it had caused the passage of an enormous number of threadworms. On this hint Burnett used Scirrhinum very successfully in the treatment of threadworms, and this has been amply confirmed ever since. When there are no clear-cut indications for such remedies as Cina, Spigelia or Sulphur, or else when the results of these or other threadworm remedies have been unsatisfactory, I have for many years prescribed Scirrhinum 200c, three doses every six hours in one day, with almost invariable success. It may have to be repeated because of re-infection, especially within the family.

Dr James Runcie found that when Carcinosin was constitutionally indicated, Scirrhinum gave satisfactory results in hypertension.

Carcinosin in the Treatment of Malignant Disease

An impressive record of treatment of cancer is to be found in a paper read to the International Homoeopathic Association in 1927, entitled 'The Cancer Problem: Some Deductions Based on Clinical Experience', by Dr R. M. Le Hunt Cooper. The basis of this approach, which was introduced by his father Dr Robert T. Cooper, was to prescribe remedies known to have an effect on disease at the site of the growth, in a mother tincture which had been exposed to sunshine for three hours in unit doses, at intervals sometimes of weeks. Ornithogalum (Star of Bethlehem) was the local remedy for stomach cancer. A reference to this is to be found in Clark's *Dictionary*. Ruta was the local remedy for cancer of the rectum, and Ruta cured one case in my experience. Mentha Pulegium (Penny Royal), extensively used in the past to cause abortion, was used in uterine cancer; Scrophularia Nosode or Belladonna for cancer of the breast; Symphytum for cancer of bone. Carcinosin was regarded as essential and was given in all cases in the thirtieth or two-hundreth potency at intervals of a week or more. The paper is illustrated by drawings and photographs.

Aggravation from the unit doses was sometimes severe and the evidence is certainly convincing. Dr Le Hunt Cooper believed in avoiding surgery if possible, but considered that radiotherapy, which in his day was by X-rays expertly given, could be effective, arguing that such therapy was essentially homoeopathic. It is unfortunate that the approach to treatment outlined in Dr Cooper's paper has not been thoroughly investigated. One of his associates, Dr George Burford, senior consultant gynaecologist to the London Homoeopathic Hospital, gave an address to the British Homoeopathic Society in January 1933 in which he described cures of eight cases of malignancy. Details of treatment were incomplete, but he gave Carcinosin to all patients as well as other remedies.

My study and experience over the past thirty years has been devoted almost exclusively to the indications and use of Carcinosins as constitutional remedies.

The following two cases treated along Dr Le Hunt Cooper's lines are interesting, although there was no positive evidence of malignancy. A woman of thirty-seven had a module about one inch in diameter in her right breast, associated with peau d'orange and moderately enlarged axillary lymph glands. There were constitutional indications for Carcinosin; and although not recorded by Dr Le Hunt Cooper, Bellis Perennis has a clinical record of success in dealing with nodules and cancer of the breast. A dose of Carcinosin 30c was followed by five drops of the mother tincture of Bellis Perennis (not exposed to sunshine) t.i.d., a.c. ex aqua was given, after which there was a slight improvement. Following two similar courses the nodule had become about a third of its original size, and the peau d'orange had disappeared. I prescribed Scirrhinum 200c, and this was followed by further improvement although a small mass remained. The axillary glands were considerably reduced in size. There was no recurrence during the following four years, after which I lost touch with her.

A woman of eighty had a very similar nodule accompanied by peau d'orange in her left breast, and almost identical treatment was given with a similar result including disappearance of the peau d'orange. There was no recurrence during the following three years.

Chapter 14

Carcinosin: Case Histories

Anal Prolapse
A man of forty complained of severe anal prolapse occurring after defaecation. The onset was associated with considerable mental stress through being unfairly treated at his work, and he had put on much weight.

Family History. His father's mother and his own father were diabetic, and his father died of cancer of the rectum.

Consideration of Treatment. Mentals and generals and local symptoms suggested consideration of Lachesis, Sepia, Natrum Mur. and Sulphur, all being remedies complementary to Carcinosin.

Treatment. This consisted of a weight-reducing diet, Folliculinum 30c followed three days later by a daily dose of Carcinosin Bowel Co. 30c for three days. This resulted in cure.

Asthma
A boy of thirteen had suffered from asthma from the age of two, both spasmodic and bronchial attacks.

Previous Illness. Three attacks of pneumonia, at three months, twelve months and eighteen months of age. Asthma started after the second pneumonia.

Family History. Nil, except tendency to asthma on father's side. Dissimilar twin brother also had asthma, for which he was given Medorrhinum, which cured him.

Mentals and Generals. Carcinosin appearance. Moles. Sensitive to reprimand. Loves fat meat. Asthma always better at the seaside.

In this case Medorrhinum seemed indicated, except for the love of fat meat – an example of two or more partial indications for related remedies. Carcinosin 200c was given and during the following year he had only two minor attacks.

Boils

A woman of thirty suffered from boils in the ears, alternating from one ear to the other. Chemotherapy helped to clear up the boils but did not stop recurrence. She had no freedom from boils for more than a week or two at a time. The following symptoms were present:

Dislikes consolation. Could not weep even when she lost her mother, who died from cancer of the uterus.
Nausea and vomiting at the beginning of her periods. Dragging down at menses.
Headache before a thunderstorm.
Tired in the morning, better in the evening.
Profuse offensive axillary perspiration.

Natrum Mur. and Gelsemium have sadness but cannot weep. Sepia however, which contains Natrum Mur., seemed to be much more indicated.

The patient was given Sepia 30c, 200c and 1M on three consecutive days. She had a week's aggravation, then six weeks freedom and her menstrual symptoms were relieved. She was then given Sepia 200c, 1M and 10M, which was followed by three weeks freedom, after which another relapse. Carcinosin 30c, 200c and 1M was given. It was followed by a severe aggravation lasting about a week and was then followed by complete freedom for three years.

Catarrh

A girl of fifteen had had a chronic yellow nasal catarrh and frequent colds practically all her life. Her condition had been worse since whooping cough at the age of eleven.

Previous History. Tonsils and adenoids removed. Measles badly. Whooping cough very badly. All childish illnesses more severe than her five siblings.

Family History. Mother died of cancer of the oesophagus.

Mentals and Generals. Timid, loves affection, chews her nails. Very fond of dancing. Terrific reader. Feels a fright in her stomach. Starts at noise. Anticipation of chlorine in a swimming bath starts up eczema. Anticipation may cause vomiting. Carcinosin appearance.

Pulsatilla and Sepia were considered, but in view of her appearance, the severe whooping cough, and the fact that both Pulsatilla and Sepia are related to Carcinosin, she was given Carcinosin Adeno. Stom. 30c, 200c and 1M, selected because of fright in the stomach and vomiting on anticipation.

There was a violent aggravation after which her catarrh and colds vanished for a year.

Colds

A boy of eight suffered from almost constant colds characterised by watery nasal discharge. He caught cold on the least exposure to chill or draughts. His schooling had been seriously curtailed.

Family History. N.A.D.

Previous Illness. Tonsils and adenoids removed, but without beneficial effect.

On Examination. Considerably underweight. This boy presented the Carcinosin appearance, blue sclerotics, moles and café-au-lait complexion. Anterior and posterior cervical glands were enlarged. Sinuses normal radiologically, otherwise N.A.D.

Mentals and Generals. His mother described him as having a gentle disposition, more like a girl than a boy, and said he had difficulty in holding his own with other boys. He was very sympathetic and craved affection. Extremely sensitive to music. He had a craving for milk and butter, and a dislike of fat meat and fat bacon.

Treatment. He was given Carcinosin 30c, 200c and 1M on three consecutive days. This was followed by a remarkable improvement, but six weeks later he fractured an arm and had to be admitted to another hospital.

When he was discharged his mother described the situation as if he were bottling up a fright. Opium CM was given with excellent effect. A week later the Carcinosin prescription was repeated. He ceased to have colds and gained nearly a stone in weight within three months of the commencement of treatment. I saw him on two occasions in the following eighteen months and he had maintained excellent health, and there was no trouble in holding his own with other boys.

Nephritis

A girl was first seen at the age of eleven, having been discharged from a teaching hospital with second-stage nephritis following a severe acute attack. The urine had 6 parts albumen per 1,000, and a few granular casts, many leucocytes and lower urinary tract epithelial cells. Blood urea 22mg per cent. This had persisted for some time and a very gloomy prognosis had been given.

Previous Illness. Whooping cough, measles, tonsillitis.

Family History. Nil.

Mentals and Generals. Typical appearance café-au-lait complexion, numerous moles, very blue sclerotics. Desires salt, eggs. Aversion to milk. Sleeps well.

Treatment. Carcinosin 30c, 200c and 1M was given, and a month later Sepia 12c.

There was a great improvement in general health – the albumen went down fairly rapidly to 1 part per 1,000 and the urine was otherwise normal. This persisted, and ten months later a dose of the bowel nosode Mutabile Patterson 200c was given. The next specimen was clear and there was no recurrence of albumen during the following year. This nosode has been effective in a number of cases of persistent urinary tract infection.

Osteoarthritis

A woman of forty-five. Generalised early osteoarthritis in hands, feet and spine.

Previous Illness. Recurrent pseudocyesis with enlarged abdomen and milk in breasts. Tubes ligated on advice of psychiatrist. Prolonged fear in childhood caused by sadistic father. Used to stammer, still cannot say certain words, including the number eight.

Family History. Nil.

Mentals and Generals. Sympathetic to others and loved affection. Sentimental. Headache in thunderstorm. Loves dancing. Sensitive to certain people. Weak ankles. Still afraid in dark. Never weeps.

Treatment. Carcinosin 30c, 200c and 1M was given with remarkable benefit, and patient could now say 'eight'. Fifteen weeks later, Sepia 12c was given, also Ruta and Iron in low potency.

Post-hysterectomy Problems

A woman of fifty-one, mother of three, complained of waking up between 2 a.m. and 4 a.m. finding her hands firmly and painfully clutched together across her chest, accompanied by hot flushes and copious sweating of head and chest. This began two years previously, after a hysterectomy on account of a uterine fibroid. She was very upset by the anaesthetic and said she had changed from being a cheerful, energetic and sympathetic person to one who was very depressed but could not weep. She was in an apathetic state, and since the operation had had outbursts of intense irritability with her husband and children. She sometimes also had a sensation as if her period was coming on, including premenstrual tension. She felt better by the seaside. Although she was aggravated by warm, wet weather and before a thunderstorm, she loved watching the lightning. She had an aversion to fat meat.

Family History. Nothing outstanding.

Past History. Hay fever. Her son was a diabetic.

Consideration of Treatment. There were strong partial indications for Lachesis and Sepia; both cover menopause, periodicity at night, worse during and after sleep, flushes of heat with sweat, menorrhagia; both affect acute and chronic hepatitis, which might relate to the effects of the anaesthesia. Lachesis covers clutching the fingers together, worse in warm wet weather, and uterine fibroids, which are not covered by Sepia. Sepia covers better at the seaside, aversion to fat meat, indifferent to loved ones at times, which is not covered by Lachesis. Carcinosin covers menopause, enjoyment watching a thunderstorm, and the important mental symptom 'Sadness but cannot weep'. It is complementary to both Lachesis and Sepia.

Treatment. Carcinosin Bowel Co. 30c was given, followed four days later by Lachesis 10M. This resulted in a break of the regular occurrence of the nightly symptoms. She felt better generally. A month later she was given Sepia five doses to be taken at five-day intervals, which was followed by considerable further improvement, and the Sepia was spread out to ten-day intervals. This was followed by complete remission of the nightly symptoms and she felt extremely well in herself.

I happened to see her four years later on account of an unrelated complaint and she reported that there had been no relapse.

Rectal Prolapse

A boy of seven had suffered from prolapse of the rectum 'practically from birth', which was premature, and according to his mother he took some weeks to recover. At eighteen months he had a severe attack of whooping cough with convulsions and took a long time to recover. The prolapse occurred with every stool and had to be pushed back.

Mentals and Generals. He was very tidy and felt much better when at the seaside.

On Examination. Considerably underweight, and he had the full Carcinosin appearance.

Treatment. On account of his slow recovery from birth, the severe attack of whooping cough at an early age, his appearance, his tidy disposition and amelioration at the seaside, a prescription of Carcinosin 200c was given. This was followed by a general improvement in health, and the prolapse occurred only occasionally. Five months later Carcinosin 200c was repeated as the improvement, although maintained, was not progressive. This resulted in complete cure.

Prolapse of the rectum in children often cures itself, but the relationship of improvement to Carcinosin in this case suggested that it played a part.

Tonic Convulsions

A woman of fifty complained of tonic convulsions starting a year after the menopause, which had occurred when she was forty-eight. The first attack was associated with a slight injury to her hand and occurred in the daytime; subsequent attacks always came on at night. She work up feeling very hot and sweaty with a great feeling of stiffness and heaviness all over, she tore the clothing off her chest and abdomen and then fell unconscious for about fifteen minutes. When she woke up she felt extremely tired. Hospital investigation was negative and her doctor was advised to put her on anti-convulsive treatment, but this was ineffective.

Consideration of Treatment. There was a strong family history of cancer and she had a head injury at the age of five. She said that her neck was still occasionally a little stiff and at times required massage.

On Examination. There was limitation of rotation of the neck.

Treatment. I gently freed the cervical spine, resulting in free rotation. From a homoeopathic point of view the family history, together with the onset coming after the menopause, suggested Carcinosin. Two other remedies related to the menopause were partly indicated: Lachesis and Sepia. Lachesis was preferable because of the pattern of onset of the attacks – after sleep – and the fact that she could not bear any clothing on her abdomen at that time. Carcinosin 30c one dose was given, followed a week later by Lachesis 10M. This was followed by a remarkable improvement although she still had an occasional attack. Lachesis 10M was given two months later. This was followed by still further improvement, and during the following year she only very occasionally had an attack. Carcinosin 30c followed a week later by Lachesis 10M was then given and this resulted in cure.

Warts

A young man of eighteen complained of warts on his face at the mucocutaneous junction of his lips and on his fingers adjacent to the nails.

Past History. Emotional insecurity related to separation of his parents. (Insecurity covered in Kent's *Repertory* by 'Homesickness'.) Had attempted suicide.

Family History. Tuberculosis and malignancy strongly represented.

Mentals and Generals. Sympathetic. Scars tend to break open.

Consideration of Treatment. Causticum, a near specific for warts at mucocutaneous junction. Warts close to nails. Causticum also covers scars which tend to break open as well as the mentals 'Sympathetic', 'Homesickness', 'Desires death', and 'Suicidal disposition'.

Treatment. Causticum 200c plussed 2, 4, 6, and 8 was given on consecutive days. This had no effect on the warts. Carcinosin 30c three doses every six hours in one day was given, which was also ineffective. I then prescribed Carcinosin combined with Causticum in the thirtieth potency, three doses every six hours in one day. This was followed by the warts falling off within a month. There was a slight recurrence of the warts the following year, and the combined remedy was repeated. The warts again cleared up and there was no recurrence during the following five years.

In a very few similar cases, I found the combined remedy was successful when apparently clear indications for a remedy failed, and where Carcinosin given separately also failed.

Chapter 15

Indications for Certain Nosodes

My interest in nosodes developed through seeing, at Dr Tyler's clinic, many cases of chronic disease, including rheumatism of various kinds, and epilepsy, clearing up rapidly under their influence. Even cancer has been modified.

Nosodes which have been proved in potency, such as Medorrhinum or Tuberculinum, when mental, general and peculiar symptoms have been brought out, can be prescribed according to the same rules which govern the prescription of other remedies. Even with these a personal or family history of infection weighs, to some extent, in their favour.

At first sight it might seem that the prescription of nosodes, unproved in potency, is made on purely pathological grounds, and not therefore in accordance with homoeopathic philosophy. The following considerations may alter that view, and show that their use as antipsorics is justified. Pathological changes can be looked on as their provings; their value in homoeoprophylaxis, and in cases such as are described below, indicate that use can be made of pathology.

Dr Samuel Swan (USA), whose work in introducing nosodes to homoeopathy is well known, says, 'Morbose poison will cure the disease which produced it, if given in high potency.' He goes on, 'Had not Hahnemann tried morbose products empirically on those sick of the disease which had produced those products, he would not have said, "Unless they were so altered by potentisation, they could never have any effect on an organism tainted with that identical virus".'

Hahnemann's doctrine of chronic diseases states that all chronic ailments are secondary manifestations of an infection or infections, acute at their inception, and later lying dormant until stimulated to flare up in the various guises of chronic ill health by adverse circumstances such as prolonged anxiety, inadequacies of diet, and so on. According to this theory, if chronic disease can be cured by Streptococcin, for example, whether we look on psora as a single infection or as comprising the various non-venereal acute infections, Streptococcin is an important remedy which deserves more consideration.

Constantine Hering regarded all epidemic fevers, as well as acute contagious disease, as psoric. He even mentioned that there was no dividing line between psoric and non-psoric diseases. In certain cases of measles, Hahnemann noted that the patient had an unusually violent attack, or that chronic ill health followed, and ascribed these occurrences to a flare-up of latent psora, affected by the stimulus of measles.

In every acute febrile disease, each victim takes on the disease in an individual way. Might it not be an individual characteristic in one patient which causes measles or whooping cough to appear more than once, or to assume a dangerous quality or be the precursor of chronic disease, whereas in another patient these illnesses are among the comparatively trivial incidents of childhood?

We can consider the use of nosodes in three respects: prophylaxis, acute disease, and chronic disease. The first two are mentioned only briefly.

Prophylaxis
There is no doubt that a train of ill health not infrequently follows the use of cowpox inoculation, designed to immunise from smallpox. There is evidence that immunity to smallpox can otherwise be achieved by homoeopathy. Dr Swan, to whom reference has been made as a pioneer in the use of nosodes, was the medical officer to an institution of two hundred patients. The Board of Health were going to vaccinate, but he decided to give Variolinum in high potency, two doses, one at night and one the next morning. In five days all the two hundred, with the exception of forty, were very ill with the usual preliminary symptoms of smallpox, while twenty-five of the number later produced smallpox pustules, some umbilicated, some purulent; however, these passed away leaving no scars, and smallpox did not fully develop in anyone. There is evidence also that children given Variolinum in potency are immune to cowpox inoculation.

Clarke, speaking of Malandrinum, says, 'Homoeopaths here have a very effectual protection against infection with smallpox and vaccination.' Burnett writes, 'Speaking for myself, I have for the last nine years been in the habit of using vaccine matter in the thirtieth homoeopathic centesimal potency whenever smallpox was about, and have, thus far, not seen anyone so treated get variola.'

Another example is seen in diphtheria prophylaxis. A procedure was successfully adopted in the children's ward of the Royal London Homoeopathic Hospital, under which contacts were given Diphtherinum

200c, one dose. Dr Lees of Dundee gave one hundred contacts of diphtheria the nosode in potency without a single case developing the disease.

These instances merely indicate the possibilities of homoeopathic prophylaxis.

Acute Disease

Nosodes are sometimes effective in clearing up lingering cases. This is discussed more fully in the chapter on 'The Significance of Past History'.

Chronic Disease

One indication of primary importance is where an acute infection marks the onset of chronic disease: 'Never well since measles', for example. My first experience with Morbillinum impressed me in that respect.

A girl of nine came with a history of having had a cough of two years duration following measles. She had been off school for most of the two years, was losing weight and was generally debilitated. Tuberculosis was suspected and she was thoroughly overhauled at one of the London teaching hospitals, by X-rays, skin tests and sputum examination, with negative results. Drosera and Carbo Veg. helped her, but Morbillinum acted like a charm. She was back at school within a month, and for the next fourteen months was able to attend school regularly. There were two slight recurrences, which did not necessitate her staying at home. Morbillinum was repeated once, six months after the first dose. She put on weight and looked extremely fit.

Another case which illustrates this is one of disseminated sclerosis. A woman of thirty-three came with a history of transient paralysis since she was eighteen years of age. She had been informed that although her condition would get better and worse, she would never completely recover. At the time of examination, in September, there was loss of sensation for heat and cold in both inferior extremities up to the inguinal region, and the knee jerks were uneven. After working out the case carefully, Causticum was prescribed with little benefit. On going into her previous illnesses, there was a history of having had a series of severe tonsillitis preceding her nervous disorder.

Streptococcin 30c, one dose, was given in October. Her symptoms cleared up in a few weeks and she was very well thereafter, except for a transient weakness in one leg the following March, which did not necessitate her staying off her work as a waitress. Streptococcin 30c, 200c, and 1M on three consecutive mornings was given, and there was no further trouble. This of course may be a natural remission, in spite of the fact that both the patient and her sister said she had never been so well since the onset of her trouble fifteen years before.

While studying this case I came across a paper by Dr Rorke, in which he gave particulars of four cases of disseminated sclerosis cured by Medorrhinum. Dr Tyler's case of cerebral tumour – a malignant endothelioma – is well known. A girl who had been in great pain for eight years, in spite of treatment and two operations on the brain at the National Hospital for Nervous Diseases, came to her outpatient clinic. It was during one of the operations that the malignant character of the growth was disclosed.

The condition commenced after a bad attack of diphtheria; she had only been given Diphtherinum 200c at long intervals. Although it is difficult to foresee the long-term result, she was completely free from pain ever since the first dose of Diphtherinum, given two years previously.

In another case, a boy of eight suffered from enuresis most of his life. He had been helped greatly by Lycopodium 200c and later, Lycopodium 10M, but was not quite cured after treatment for ten months. At the age of two he had had diphtheria very badly, being ill for eight months. Diphtherinum 200c was given. Seven months later he was discharged from the outpatients' department as cured.

The second general indication is in a patient who has had an interval of good health preceded by either severe or repeated acute infection, prior to the onset of chronic disease.

A woman of seventy-eight had suffered from cardiac disease for over twenty years. The pulse showed an irregularity on three occasions when I examined her. The only acute illness she knew about was measles, which she had had very badly. Morbillinum 30c, one dose, was given. Within a week the pulse was restored to normal rhythm and she was decidedly benefited in strength and appearance.

Many of the streptococcal cases have a history of one outstanding acute illness, sometimes repeated. The majority of patients have had several childish ailments, and it is only by questioning carefully that one gets the history into perspective.

It seems probable that the first lapse from health is important, in the same way that vaccination may be the basis on which chronic ill-health rests.

A woman of forty-two came complaining of feeling generally unfit. She suffered from frequent headaches and flatulent dyspepsia, which had troubled her for eighteen years, following an attack of jaundice. An unusually long list of acute illnesses was given. She had been very healthy up to the time she had measles at the age of three. Morbillinum was given with marked benefit in general health, and the headaches ceased. Flatulence was helped later by Carbo Veg.

A case of migraine was greatly improved by Morbillinum, which was the simillimum to her first illness which she had had slightly, although Diphtherinum, given on a history of having almost died from diphtheria, had no appreciable effect.

The third indication may be termed the pathological indication. Each acute infection selects certain tissues for its chief manifestation, although the boundaries of each domain are vaguely defined and overlap one another.

The most common indications are tonsillitis, severe or repeated, or else repeated quinsies. The various well-known manifestations of acute rheumatism follow. The mental depression caused by the activity of streptococcal infection in chronic cases has also been noted.

On analysing a number of streptococcal cases, to find if there were any other common features, I found that in more than half the cases the following mental symptom was present: 'Sympathy causes weeping'. If such a patient was asked, 'What effect does sympathy have on you?' she would immediately reply, 'It makes me weep.' I have seen this in over ten cases. 'Better from sea air' is also a common symptom.

Although the number of cases is too small to make the analysis of much value, the relationship of Sulphur to streptococcal infection and to Streptococcin was confirmed. One case was helped by Sulphur 10M and later by Sulphur CM, and still later by Streptococcin. Sulphur – the great anti-psoric!

The relationship of Pyrogen, which contains a number of strains of streptococci, was also apparently confirmed in a few cases, where a mouthful of carious teeth were removed prior to onset of the trouble. The indication and the history of ill-health following abortion of labour, where no pelvic pathology can be detected, has been well proved in practice as an indication for Pyrogen.

Boericke gives Arnica as being related to streptococcal infection – Arnica with its clinical record of successful administration after labour, and in heart cases.

Scarlatinum clears up some cases dating from scarlet fever. For example, a woman who had suffered from an itching erythematous, papular and vesicular eruption for eight years, responded rapidly to Scarlatinum. Some cases are responsive to Streptococcin where Scarlatinum fails.

A case of rheumatoid arthritis came to Dr Tyler's outpatients after eight years of trouble. Both wrists were fixed. The knuckles were involved and ulnar deviation was present. The right hand could, with difficulty, be brought to the level of the nose, on bending her head forward. This patient had many years of treatment. Psorinum helped on many occasions. Many years later, Streptococcin 200c, three doses, was given. Two months afterwards the patient felt very well, and Sac. Lac. was prescribed. A further four months later – 'very much better', 'does a lot of work with her hands, including cooking and washing'.

Chapter 16

Alumina

Dr R. M. Le Hunt Cooper made an extensive study of aluminium as a result of personal sensitivity to food or drink heated in aluminium utensils. Among his papers is an outline of aluminium pathogenesis published in the *British Homoeopathic Journal* in May 1942, which is well worth reading.

Another valuable contribution which includes quotations from other authorities, is to be found in Dr Tyler's *Homoeopathic Drug Pictures*. Experience has led me to decide that Alumina is rarely indicated as a main constitutional remedy. Even a superficial look through Kent's *Repertory* will show its widespread effect on man. Avoiding aluminium cooking utensils may be important to ensure the effect of other consitutional remedies, when sensitivity is indicated by certain symptoms.

It is impossible to summarise Alumina, but the following very incomplete list of symptoms can suggest looking into this question.

Itchy Eyes
Alumina causes various eye symptoms, but the most important, and not uncommon, is itching, especially of the inner canthi.

Diseases of the Alimentary Tract
From gingivitis, just occasionally, to constipation and pruritis ani.

Weakness of the Oesophageal Muscles
This can result in slowness in eating, and sometimes a sensation as if a bolus of food was stopped on the way down to the stomach.

Constipation
Constipation of various kinds may be present. A characteristic symptom is that of weakness of the rectal muscles, resulting in having to strain considerably in order to pass a stool of normal consistency. In a busy outpatient's children's clinic it is worthwhile to ask the mother if the

child rubs its eyes often, whether he is a slow eater, or if he takes a long time on the toilet. Mental symptoms are vast and varied, but in a child, obstinacy suggests consideration of sensitivity to aluminium, and Tuberculinum as a constitutional remedy if the obstinacy is very marked.

Allergic Conditions

These also call for consideration of aluminium sensitivity. When there are excessively itching skin eruptions requiring scratching, to the extent that the area becomes raw or bleeds, this is a strong indication of aluminium sensitivity.

There are two reasons for considering aluminium sensitivity in cases of migraine. Not only can Alumina cause a wide variety of head pains, but there is also the allergic component to this problem.

When aluminium sensitivity is present, it can almost always be dealt with by avoiding heating food or drink in aluminium utensils at home. Occasional contacts outside rarely matter, but if so this can be antidoted. Food or drink should be heated entirely in utensils of stainless steel, enamel, tin, iron or pyrex, and all other cooking utensils should be discarded. Care should also be taken to notice that additions to these utensils such as lids, spouts etc, are not made of aluminium. Eggs boiled in an aluminium pan absorb aluminium, and this has been demonstrated by analysis. Tin foil should not be used for oven dishes. After this procedure Alumina 30c or 200c, three doses every six or twelve hours, can be given, and constitutional treatment can be started a few days after this. Later on, should there be a relapse, this may be traced to the reintroduction of aluminium utensils, or excess exposure to outside sources, which can be antidoted.

Regarding children, it is worthwhile to tell the mother what symptoms to look for, rather than advise the child, for obvious reasons, and to supply her with Alumina 30c tablets, one to be given dry on the tongue when required, at intervals of not less than three weeks.

Chapter 17

Bellis Perennis

Arnica and Sepia share certain symptoms with Bellis Perennis, which has been comparatively neglected. Bellis Perennis has been used for the shock of falling into cold water when over-heated – there are many examples in the literature, and I have found this effective both in the UK and in India.

A record of proving of Bellis Perennis is to be found in Anshultz's *New, Old, and Forgotten Remedies*. Tyler's *Drug Pictures* gives valuable information, including reference to herbal literature and Compton Burnett's extensive experience of treatment with low potencies or mother tinctures. Dr Dorothy Shepherd's book *A Physician's Posy* is also important, providing further confirmation of Burnett's success in the treatment of tumours following injury, as well as of her own experience in dealing with prolapse of the uterus. Clarke's *Dictionary* also has a chapter on Bellis Perennis.

Bellis Perennis has long had a reputation for being superior in the treatment of soft tissue injury. In major operations I used Arnica along with Staphysagria pre- and post-operatively for many years – Staphysagria for its remarkable effect in dealing with pain in a cut wound. I changed to Bellis Perennis with Staphysagria, and so far as I can judge this was an improvement. I found the treatment to be very effective in appendicectomy, cholecystectomy, hysterectomy, herniotomy, haemorrhoidal operations and circumcisions. After-effects of head injury and/or spinal injury respond well to Bellis Perennis, whether or not it is superior to Arnica Montana. When Sepia symptoms predominate I have used this on a number of occasions.

Dr A. H. Grimmer read a paper to be found in the *Homoeopathic Recorder* entitled 'Further Results in Homoeopathic Treatment of Cancer', relating to two hundred and seventy-five cases treated by homoeopathy and diet, of which one hundred and sixty were alive after six years. The diet was not specified, but included avoiding food cooked in aluminium utensils in cancer of the alimentary tract. In the discussion,

Dr Boger described the case of a middle-aged woman whose mother had died of cancer of the breast. The woman had come to see Dr.Boger six years after having a mastectomy, complaining of pain in the scar and a lump in the axilla. After two doses of Bellis Perennis 30c were given at an interval of two weeks the lump disappeared and the pain in the scar had gone. In reply, Dr Grimmer said that Bellis Perennis has given us as many cures of cancer of the breast as any other one remedy. If you get the specific history of following an injury, it competes with Conium. In Conium the breast is apt to be painless, whereas Bellis Perennis has more or less pain.

Two women took part in the proving; one had previously had a hysterectomy and the other started taking Bellis Perennis mother tincture the day before menstruation, and the proving ran over two periods. The uterus seemed sore as if squeezed. The pain extended down the anterior aspect of the thigh during each period. No change in the character of the flow could be determined. Accompanying these symptoms were dizziness and vertigo, worse on rising up and relieved by lying down. Sepia covers cramping pain in the uterus during menstruation, and pain in the uterus extending downwards but not specifically in the anterior aspects, a difference which I have found useful in the treatment of dysmenorrhea.

Bellis Perennis has been recommended as capable of dealing with what may be called 'pus dammed up', when aggravated by heat and relieved by cold. Apical abscess seemed a safe situation in which to test this out. Arnica covers abscess of the gums and Sepia covers pain in the teeth biting them together. I found Bellis Perennis 30c t.i.d. four days, b.d. three days relieved the pain. Two had to have a short course afterwards, but out of the ten cases nine were completely relieved. I treated a few cases in a similar way giving Pyrogen and Bellis Perennis, and these also cleared up.

Dysmenorrhoea (1)

A woman of forty-one complained of dysmenorrhoea almost since puberty. It was preceded by swelling and pain in the breasts and only gradually subsided during the flow, which started ten to fourteen days after onset of mammary pain. Flow was scanty and accompanied by cramping and dragging-down pain extending down the thighs, especially anteriorly. Vulva felt as if pressed out from within, although no sign of prolapse, backache also in the lumbosacral region.

Past History. Mother three and a half days in labour. Eczema when

119

weaned at four months. Another head injury at four years. Tonsils removed. Appendicectomy. Rheumatic fever.

During Pregnancy. Morning sickness for five months. Labour induced on account of hypertension, and for this reason full anaesthesia was not given. She suffered greatly and was utterly exhausted. Was able to breast feed for six weeks only.

Mentals and Generals. Tends to become extremely depressed at times. Easily upset and angry from any injustice. Can be detached from loved ones and easily irritated by them. Sympathy to others. Fastidious. Anxiety felt in stomach. Dislikes thundery weather and snow air. Offensive sweating. Craves salt.

Sepia covers scanty periods. Pain in uterus bearing down as if everything would come out. Pain in uterus extending downwards. Pain in vagina. It also covers head injury at birth and four years of age. Fastidious and sympathetic (although neither are listed in Kent). Indifference to loved ones. Worse on approach of a thunderstorm. Worse in snow air. Anxiety felt in stomach.

Sepia is not recorded in craving for salt or in pain in breasts associated with menstruation.

Treatment. Before treatment was decided the patient developed an apical abscess, for which I prescribed Bellis Perennis 30c t.i.d. four days, b.d. three days. Menstruation occurred during this course of treatment and she found a marked freedom from mammary and uterine pain, Bellis dealing effectively with the apical abscess.

Bellis Perennis 30c was then prescribed to be taken during menstruation four-hourly first day, t.i.d. for three days or as required, and this reduced the pain considerably. Gradually a dose occasionally was all that was required.

A year later Carcinosin Bowel Co. 200c, one dose, was given as a constitutional remedy based on family history and partial indications for Sepia. This resulted in still further progress and still less need for Bellis, one dose of which was only rarely required and eventually not at all.

Dysmenorrhoea (2)

A woman of thirty-eight complained of dysmenorrhoea. Menses occurred at three to three and a half week intervals, preceded by pain in the left breast in the mid cycle, aggravated a few days before menstruation and then accompanied by a dragging-down feeling in the abdomen.

When the flow started this was replaced by cramping, bearing-down pain in the pelvis, extending down the anterior aspect of the right thigh. The pain was relieved by physical exertion.

Past History. Eczema alternating with asthma. Tonsils and adenoids removed as a child. Pneumonia at thirteen. Glandular fever at eighteen.

Family History. Mother's brother had cancer, and mother's sister had diabetes.

Mentals and Generals. Alternating moods, cheerful alternating with depression. Worried about trifles. Although not applicable in this case, 'Cheerful alternating with sadness' is the only one available to cover schizophrenia of the manic depressive type in Kent's *Repertory*. She was afraid in a thunderstorm. Very sensitive to music. Better generally at the seaside. Dry skin. Tendency to car and sea-sickness.

Sepia covers alternating moods. Fear of a storm. Sensitive to music. Better for sea air. Better for physical exertion generally, as well as during menstruation. Sepia also covers menstruation, frequent pain bearing down in abdomen before menstruation, pain cramping and bearing down at the period. Pain in the uterus extending downwards. Pain relieved by physical exertion.

Sepia does not cover the breast pain, which was quite marked, or the extension of the uterus pain down the anterior aspect of the right thigh. Bellis Perennis, which is remarkably similar to Sepia, covers both these symptoms.

Treatment. Although it is said to be inadvisable to prescribe two very similar remedies together, as there is a risk of one antidoting the other, I prescribed Bellis Perennis combined with Sepia 12c to be commenced a day or so before menstruation, given every three hours on the first day, every four hours the second day, then every six hours during the period. In such circumstances I advise taking an occasional dose during the night if in pain. This provided very considerable relief, and after a few months I omitted the Sepia from the prescription and continued with Bellis alone. This led to further improvement to the extent that I advised taking only an occasional dose when required.

In view of the family history and the episode of glandular fever, her sensitivity to music, amelioration at the seaside and the complementary relationship of Sepia and Bellis to Carcinosin, I gave a dose of Carcinosin Bowel Co. 200c. This was followed by the need for a very occasional dose of Bellis and eventually none at all.

After-effects of Injury

A man of fifty-five complained of backache, which he said he had suffered from all his life. Pain and stiffness in the cervical, upper dorsal, lumbar region, sacro-iliac joints; worse on rising in the morning and better for subsequent movement. At times sudden pains in the spine. Painful locking of the spine when turning over in bed.

Past History. Head injury at age seven, details of which were unknown.

Family History. Not known. The patient was brought up in an orphanage.

On Examination. Generally fit. Scar in region of left parieto-occipital junction. There was considerable general limitation of spinal movement on account of pain.

Mentals and Generals. Backache when mentally upset. Always a very poor memory, forgets what he has just read, or intended to do. Intensely interested in classical music, plays records whenever there is an opportunity in daytime or evening. Can be indifferent to loved ones. In himself is very much better at the seaside and intensely dislikes warm weather. Strongly averse to fat meat. Sweats very easily on slight exertion, especially the feet.

Treatment. Gentle manipulation to free spine. Seen two weeks later and reported that he could now turn over in bed without pain, but the other pains were as before.

Consideration of Homoeopathic Prescription. Head injury with scar, together with his type of memory and his ability to become detached from loved ones strongly suggested Helleborus and Sepia. Sepia covers sensitivity to music, better at the seaside. Backache when beginning to move and better for subsequent movement. Sudden pain in the back may be covered by Sepia, one description is 'As if hit on the spine by a hammer', and Sepia is the only remedy recorded. Perspiration on slight exertion, Sepia in black type; Helleborus also covers aversion to fat meat, and Sepia is worse in cold weather. Sepia could probably have helped in this case, but Bellis Perennis seemed preferable because of the severe head injury and also the dislike of warm weather. Although complaints of Bellis Perennis may typically come on after a ducking in cold water when overheated, Bellis Perennis patients are very often worse from heat. Sepia patients are almost always worse in cold weather.

I gave him Bellis Perennis 30c combined with Helleborus 30c plussed 2, 4, and 6 on consecutive days, and Rhus Tox. liniment to be applied daily in the spinal muscles. Three weeks later he was generally very much better and was given placebo. A month later I had a letter saying, 'I am really very much better and would like to cancel my appointment, thank you so much for all your help.' A report a year later said, 'Only occasional slight backache, no need for further treatment.'

This case illustrates the way in which Helleborus can be combined with another member of the group of remedies having an effect on head injuries, and some points of the relationship between Bellis Perennis and Sepia.

Rheumatism

A man aged forty.

Complaint. Pain in both legs, drawing, cramping, heaviness when walking on pavement.

Onset. After getting thoroughly wet and cold when over-heated playing golf, two years previously.

Previous Illnesses. Measles affecting eyes, and had to wear glasses since then. Many injuries, mainly head and spine from rugby football which he enjoyed from the age of eight to twenty-six, when he turned to golf.

On Examination. Generally fit. Movement of knees and ankles free and painless. In this case the mode of onset, becoming cold and wet when over-heated, together with his many injuries of the past, suggests Bellis.

Sepia was indicated on the following grounds:

1) Patient was always better from physical exertion. He took up golf when the effects of multiple injuries stopped him playing rugger. (See Kent's *Repertory* in Generalities, 'Exertion ameliorates'.)

2) He perspired profusely in the axillae, a symptom not so commonly found in the male and which may be considered outside the norm.

3) Sympathetic to others. He worked for a local authority and this entailed advising members of the community on their problems; he said he found it very difficult not to become involved. When I asked him if he was often asked advice outside his work, he replied quickly, 'Very often'. As always, one must be on one's guard when asking questions. The vehemence and quickness of the reply influence the assessment as to whether the symptom can be part of the basis on which the individual prescription is made. (Sometimes one can be helped in making an assessment from information derived from relatives or intimate associates.) If there is any doubt about a symptom, it should be discarded for this purpose.

4) Sepia covers in general, heavy lower limbs, cramping in lower limbs, and drawing pains in legs, but does not in Kent's *Repertory* cover worse for jarring. Sepia is however in black type in Generalities, 'Worse for jarring'.

5) Fear in high places. Afraid of going near edge of sea cliffs and when climbing a ladder. Sepia has vertigo looking down.

6) Loves watching a thunderstorm. His wife told me that he had to open the tent door to watch the lightning while on a camping holiday. Sepia is the only remedy recorded for this symptom, but in my experience Bellis Perennis and Carcinosin can be added.

Bellis Perennis 30c, 200c, 1M on consecutive days was given. This relieved the pains completely and his wife said that he was no longer afraid when climbing a ladder, and there was much less fear when walking near cliffs. No further treatment was given until a year and a half later, when he said that there had been a slight return of pain in the legs, at which point I repeated the prescription.

This case illustrates the importance of the onset of an illness resulting from sudden exposure to cold and wet. Also, the history of many injuries together with Sepia symptoms including 'Sympathetic to others, better for exertion, aggravation from jarring, and enjoyment from watching a thunderstorm'.

Chapter 18

Folliculinum: A Synthetic Oestrogen

This remedy has not been proved, but it is a very useful addition to the materia medica.

From birth onwards restrictions of various kinds are imposed by the behaviour of others. It is when reaction to such imposition, past or present, can be judged to be well outside the norm that Folliculinum should be considered. For example, an upbringing judged to be overstrict, including well-intended stress on religion; a child having undue difficulty in standing up to aggression of others or to school discipline; undue anxiety about exams when the child feels that he is loved for his achievements rather than for himself. Later on, undue control by relatives may be a factor. It is well known that a broken home may cause insecurity.

A middle-aged woman was awakened frequently at night by a neurotic mother who used to come into her room, thus frightening her. The mother also controlled her financially. It seemed unlikely that much could be done about this, but Folliculinum 30c three times a day for three days resulted in complete abolition of this anxiety.

Undue reaction to superiors at work, whether civilian or in the armed forces; for example, being bullied or refused what seems to be deserved promotion are situations in which Folliculinum should also be considered. Over several years I have found that Folliculinum 30c works well, given three or four days before an individually-selected constitutional remedy. The two most commonly indicated constitutional remedies in such cases have been Carcinosin or Sepia, but there are others. Limited experience of Folliculinum in cases of itching skin eruptions has led to its discontinuance because of severe aggravation.

Occasionally self-imposed control comes into the picture, as the following example illustrates. A district nurse complained of chronic sore throat, the pain alternating from side to side. Devoted to her parents, she had nursed her father until he died, and then her mother. During this time she had given up an opportunity of marriage and felt depressed and frustrated. Sepia covered these symptoms, emotional insecurity and frustration listed in Kent as 'Homesickness' and 'Mortification'. Sepia 30c t.i.d. three days was given without effect. Carcinosin 20c was next prescribed on family history, her mental state, and because it is complementary to Sepia; Carcinosin also covers symptoms alternating from side to side, in my experience, but it also failed. In this case, self-imposed control suggested consideration of Folliculinum. I prescribed Folliculinum 30c followed a week later by Sepia 30c t.i.d. three days. This was followed by complete cure lasting for about six months, after which there was a slight relapse. I repeated the prescription resulting in long-lasting relief.

Chapter 19

Helleborus Niger

In a preface to the provings of Helleborus, Hahnemann wrote: 'The symptoms which I and some of my disciples have observed from the root are but few in number: still they constitute a commencement of the investigation of its properties. They serve to show that Helleborus must prove useful in a peculiar kind of fever, some dropsical affections and mental derangements.'

Among the contributions to homoeopathy made by Dr Royal Hayes is a paper published in the *Homoeopathic Recorder* in December 1948. This paper describes a series of cases illustrating the value of Helleborus in dealing with the after-effects of head injury. Helleborus is not listed in Kent's *Repertory* giving the main remedies found to be useful in the treatment of such patients: Arnica, Cicuta, Natrum Mur. and Natrum Sulph. Nor is it given in the other rubric: 'Pain, Mechanical injuries, After'. Helleborus is to be found in second type in the rubric on concussion, reflecting the view that the post-concussion syndrome consisting of headache, dizziness, forgetfulness, personality changes, difficulty in concentration and maybe insomnia, was a clinical entity separate from the after-effects of head injury in patients who had not suffered from concussion. Recent research has shown that the two conditions cannot be distinguished on this basis, i.e. on the presence or absence of a history of concussion. The rubrics on head injury can therefore be combined with the one on concussion, and for practical purposes Helleborus can thus be added to the commonly indicated head injury remedies – those given above – although obviously this does not eliminate other remedies in every case.

Since reading this paper by Dr Royal Hayes I have often used Helleborus, either on its own indications or, as not infrequently happens, when there are no apparently clear indications for anything else, and the results have been surprisingly good. Helleborus seems to be specially required when there is a history of severe concussion. Helleborus should also be considered when there is a history of head injury in the distant past, including a history or clinical evidence of a birth or prenatal injury. Naturally in such cases other head injury remedies must be compared, but when no clear indications emerge, Helleborus is worth a trial.

Hahnemann mentions mental derangement. To give an example, I found that Helleborus had a dramatic effect in a case of schizophrenia, in a patient who had not previously obtained benefit from drugs and ECT, who had had concussion several years before his illness started. Marked features were lack of concentration in a man who had had a brilliant academic and professional career, and extreme forgetfulness – forgot what he had just done and could not remember what he was about to do – strongly marked symptoms of Helleborus. Helleborus 1M plussed to six was given at first, as higher potencies may have a decided aggravation, and after two courses of this he was given the 10M. In a period of eight months he recovered completely.

Chapter 20

Lac Caninum

Kent suggested that all the milks should be fully proved, as he considered they were potentially remedies of great value. Lac Caninum was first proved one hundred and twenty years ago, in the 30th and 200th potencies. A good account of the original provings and some clinical verifications are to be found in Swan's *Materia Medica*.

Two features of Lac Caninum are well known: the tendency for complaints to shift from one side of the body to the other and back again, a strongly verified characteristic, and dreams or visions of snakes, make one immediately think of it. It is perhaps because these symptoms are so dramatic and peculiar that other pointers to Lac Caninum are sometimes missed.

Mentals

Loss of memory may be very marked. The type of forgetfulness being exemplified by the woman who goes into a shop, forgets what she came for, or having purchased something walks away without it. Absent-mindedness. There may be mental confusion, inability to concentrate, a dazed feeling and a sense of unreality. Allen stresses the use of Lac Caninum in highly sensitive, anxious, restless patients. It can produce intense irritability and hatred of everything and everybody, or the deepest despair, and it is full of fear, including fear of death and fear of disease, for example of consumption or cancer. There are visions of other horrible things besides snakes, and a delusion 'as if she were a loathsome mass of disease' is a clinically verified symptom. Other remedies immediately come to mind for these symptoms and Lac Caninum can be missed.

As well as the dreams of snakes, a number of the provers had dreams of eating. A careful study of the mental symptoms will show that Lac Caninum may fit many cases of psychoneurosis and even psychoses.

Before briefly describing a case of this sort it is hardly necessary to say that the cases to be mentioned or quoted in more length are not intended to be put forward as proofs of the action of Lac Caninum but merely to illustrate the type of case in which it has been found useful. Obviously in any single case there could be no absolute assurance that the cure was the result of one or more remedies.

A woman of 34 developed an obsession for washing herself in disinfectants, which began as an attempt to avoid infection by cancer from which her mother had died five years previously. She had convulsive treatment before homoeopathy, but this did not help. Lueticum and Ignatia were given and she was slightly improved. Her memory was very poor, especially for events before the convulsive therapy, and she used wrong words. There was a craving for salt. Lac Caninum 200c and later 10M were given with great benefit. Lueticum was given again, and she came back to her doctor a few months later because of an injury, stating that she had had no return of her previous complaint. This illustrates the use of Lac Caninum in mental diseases.

Vertigo
Under this heading a sensation of floating in the air occurs.

A curious kind of vertigo disturbed some of the provers, a sensation as if the bed were moving under them. Recently, what was probably an involuntary proving occurred. I quote from a letter from the doctor concerned: 'A few months ago I was making up some powders of Lac Caninum 30c, and I think I got some on my fingers and accidentally touched my mouth. That was about 8 p.m. and I went to bed as usual at about 11 p.m. I got quite a shock when lying down – the end of the bed under my head suddenly appeared to sink away. I could not account for it. Next day I drove my car round as usual but did not feel steady; in the evening I had difficulty in walking straight, and my daughter sent for a doctor I know. He went over me: BP all right, nothing to find. He said I had been overworking! The following day I felt more steady and within three days all the unsteadiness had gone. On looking up Lac Caninum I came to the conclusion it was the cause of the trouble.'

Head
Some provers had pains alternating from side to side, and similar headaches have been cured by Lac Caninum. Many provers had unilateral or frontal headaches, or headaches starting in the nape of the neck or occiput and coming forward over the head to settle over one or other eye. Neuralgic headaches, throbbing headaches, pressure on the vertex, and stitching or cutting pains may be present. Stitching or darting pains are incidentally found in many places. The provings suggest a use in

migraine, for which Lac Caninum has a clinical reputation. In Kent's *Lesser Writings* a case of sick headache is recorded in which Lac Caninum and Sulphur were given with improvement, Lac Caninum being used to complete the cure. Two cases of periodic headache with blurred vision were cured by Lac Caninum, the symptom which led to its consideration being a desire for pepper. It is the only remedy with that symptom. Excessive dandruff and very sensitive sores on the scalp may occur.

In conditions of the eyes, nose and ears, alternation of symptoms most commonly suggests this remedy. Stitching pains are also to be found here.

Eye
One of the historic uses of Lac Caninum is in diseases of the eye. The sensation of a film over the eye was found repeatedly. A peculiar symptom relating to sight is that visual impressions tend to be retained longer than usual on the retina. Cases of corneal ulceration and acute conjunctivitis and styes, the symptoms changing from one side to the other, have been cured. One case of corneal ulceration which had resisted specialist treatment for ten years was cured by Lac Caninum.

Nose
In the nose there is a tendency for sores to appear in the nostrils, and for acrid or bland discharges shifting from side to side. Sometimes there is alternation of stuffing-up of one side of the nose and the other. Clinically, coryzas and chronic nasal catarrh have been benefited by Lac Caninum.

Throat
The throat is especially affected. Allen states, 'Probably no remedy in the materia medica presents a more valuable pathogenesis in symptoms of the throat or one that will repay a careful study.' Sore throats may begin with itching, tingling and dryness, sometimes causing a cough. Sensations of constriction or tightness or stiffness of the throat are common. The mucous membrane of the throat feels raw or sore, again sometimes with sharp pains. Sensation of a lump on one side of the throat is a common symptom, often associated with a constant inclination to swallow, which is often extremely painful. Worse for empty swallowing, sometimes. Sore throats coinciding with menstruation is a link with the effect of Lac Caninum on the endocrine system.

The alternation of symptoms from side to side, most commonly beginning on the right side, is very well known. Here you get the strongly suggestive combination of a peculiar modality and a site of election. The cervical glands may enlarge and subside on the affected side, as might be expected. Any of the mental states of Lac Caninum may be present, including dreams of snakes. There may be frequency of micturition and frequent urging to stool. Prostration may be very marked. There may be profuse sweat which may stain the clothing brown. Warm or cold drinks may be desired, or the patient may complain of thirst but is afraid to drink. The face may be red or pale, or alternately red and pale. It may be red on one side. Most Lac Caninum throats are painful, but occasionally pain is strikingly absent.

It is a remedy for foul throats with offensive breaths. The appearance is often of great value; typically there is a milky white exudate on the tonsil or, as in the case of diphtheria, extending beyond the faucial pillars. The back of the tongue may also have a milky white coating. The exudate and tongue may be discoloured grey or yellow, or green, or even black. Small irregular ulcers may be present, and as well as alternation of sides there may be totally irregular coming and going of patches or inflammation or ulceration. This irregular shifting of symptoms is almost as equally marked in Lac Caninum as alternation of symptoms. The throat may be devoid of exudate and present a glazed appearance, either pale or red. It may be intensely red and congested, or pale with red streaks. This glazed appearance may be found in ulcers elsewhere, and is characteristic.

Lac Caninum has a clinical record in cases of diphtheria, acute and subacute tonsillitis, quinsy and even syphilitic throat manifestations. Attention is most commonly drawn to Lac Caninum when the symptoms change from one side to the other and often after the condition has persisted for some time. The appearance of the throat, however, may be so characteristic that it may be the initial pointer.

In one case the throat was very red and congested, there were milky white patches on the tonsils, and the uvula, which was more than twice its normal size, presented a mottled red and white appearance. The posterior half of the tongue was also coated milky white. The neck felt stiff but there was a surprising absence of pain. The infection cleared up very rapidly on Lac Caninum.

When we think of the various kinds of infection of the throat influenced by Lac Caninum, or for that matter by any other homoeo-pathically chosen remedy, we cannot help being impressed by the fundamental soundness of homoeopathy as compared with chemo-therapy. As it is at present, chemotherapy is ultimately bound to fail, because of the multiplication of non-sensitive organisms.

Diphtheria

Prophylaxis

There are some interesting aspects of this remedy in relation to diphtheria. It has been frequently given as a prophylatic and great success claimed. We are sometimes asked for advice as to whether or not a child should be immunised against diphtheria. Statistics clearly indicate that it is an effective safeguard and that should diphtheria occur it is seldom fatal. How does the use of Lac Caninum or Diphtherinum or Merc. Cyanide compare? We really do not know, but surely we would be comparing essentially different methods of prophylaxis. Diphtheria immunisation gives the body a training in dealing with diphtheria. If we give a remedy in potency as a prophylatic during an epidemic, it seems to me that we do so with the idea that it lingers in the body. Should infection occur, it has the same effect as if it were given at the exact moment of the onset of the disease. There is no doubt that Lac Caninum would be effective in epidemics when the symptoms of the disease in that epidemic were similar to Lac Caninum, but is it sufficiently similar to all cases of diphtheria to be always effective as a prophylatic in any epidemic?

There is another point to be kept in mind. In the UK only a very small percentage of diphtheria cases get homoeopathic treatment. Are we right in advising against a proven method of prophylaxis, and depriving the child, possibly, of any protection at all? I personally advise that the child should be immunised and during an epidemic given Diphtherinum 200c at weekly or two-weekly intervals, or more often if in actual contact with a case of diphtheria. If the genus epidemicus corresponded to Lac Caninum or any other remedy, that remedy could be used instead.

Diphtheria immunisation is not without after-effects in some cases, such as paresis or a tendency to fall, etc. These effects can be dealt with homoeopathically. It has been stated that Lac Caninum bears the same relationship to the Schick test that Thuja bears to vaccination, and it is, therefore, to be kept in mind in these occasional cases in which diphtheria immunisation has proved harmful.

Treatment

Shortly after it was originally potentised, Lac Caninum was used with great success in an epidemic of diphtheria in New York. Merc. Cyanide also has a fine record in the treatment of diphtheria. It is unfortunate that we have so little opportunity of using homoeopathy in this disease, but it responds sometimes so quickly that the initial dose or two given before the child is removed to a fever hospital may cause the diagnosis to be queried. Serum combined with skilled treatment, if given early, seems to give extremely good results. If we were to compare a series of cases treated both ways the ability of the prescriber must be taken into account. The ideal method would be to have access to homoeopathy and serum.

There seems little doubt that complications such as paralysis would be reduced by homoeopathic treatment as they are in the other acute infections. Cases are quoted in which homoeopathic treatment has had dramatic effects on diphtheritic paralysis. These cases are not, however, suitable ones to cite as examples of homoeopathy, as it is characteristic of diphtheritic paralysis to clear up without treatment provided the patient is kept alive.

Lac Caninum is to be remembered in chronic conditions in which there has been a history of throat infection including diphtheria in the past. An example of this is given in Allen's *Materia Medica of the Nosodes*.

R.G. aged 45, married 10 years, no children. Had been impotent for six years. Had been given homoeopathic treatment for eighteen months, but the only result was that he took cold less frequently. On the advice of his doctor he visited Dr Adolph Lippe, who wrote as follows: 'I find that your patient had diphtheria about ten years ago, and was treated with inappropriate mercurials and gargles. The character of the attack was that it went from one side to the other and finally back again to the original side. Great weakness, almost paralytic, followed the attack, and he thinks he has never regained his full vigour and usual strength since this illness. I have given him a dose of Lac Caninum CM, which may be required to be followed by a dose of Pulsatilla.'

Dr A. P. Wesselhoeft, the patient's doctor, adds: 'Suffice it to say that my patient never needed the suggested dose of Pulsatilla. In three months after his visit to Philadelphia his wife was pregnant. She had since borne two remarkably healthy children.' Dr Wesselhoeft adds: 'As far as we know, Lac Caninum has no sexual weakness. That fact disturbed Dr Lippe very little in his selection. He looked deeper and found the cause and the remedy. This is true homoeopathic pathology. All the knowledge in the world of the special pathology of this case could not have revealed the remedy to anyone.'

Rheumatic Fever

To consider another aspect of throat infection, it is now generally accepted that rheumatic fever is an allergic manifestation of streptococcal infection. Recently a case of rheumatic fever responded very satisfactorily to Lac Caninum, prescribed because it was noted that the pains alternated daily from side to side. When one remembers that irregularly shifting pains are also strongly marked in this remedy, and that a clue may be given by the symptoms of the throat infection, it is possible that Lac Caninum may be found to be indicated more frequently. The pains are generally worse for motion.

Chronic Rheumatic Disease

In chronic rheumatism Lac Caninum is not infrequently indicated. A man of 60 with stiffness and pain in his spine from the cervical region to the sacrum, who showed on X-ray a mixed picture of rheumatoid and osteo-arthritis of the vertebral joints, responded extremely well to the remedy. The symptom which led to this prescription was twinges of pain alternating from one shoulder joint to the other. These joints were not affected radiologically. There was a remarkable change in this man. In addition to relief from pain he straightened up and the colour returned to his cheeks. He looked years younger.

The spine is a special region of Lac Caninum. It may be very sensitive to touch. Pains may be relieved by dorsiflexion. Lumbago with Rhus Tox. modalities (stiffness on first moving and relief from subsequent motion) has been cured by Lac Caninum. Lumbago and right-sided sciatica, associated with sore throats, have also responded. In the back there may be sharp pains under one or other scapula. There may be pains in the chest also, anteriorly, at the level of the fourth rib on either side. Pains in the back and limbs may be sharp or bruised, there may be stiffness or lameness. It has cured the effects of injuries. It affects the wrists and knees.

One case which had responded to various potencies of Ruta – a very chronic case of rheumatism – had much greater relief from Lac Caninum.

A man of 35 who had suffered from severe streptococcal throat infection while in the army developed rheumatism afterwards. The pains, which he described as 'darting twinges', shifted irregularly from joint to joint involving especially the elbows, knees and shoulder. The pains lasted a few hours to a day in each locality. On questioning it was found that the throat symptoms alternated from side to side. Lac Caninum has greatly benefited this man, but he will probably require tonsillectomy to prevent relapses.

Acute Nephritis

Acute nephritis is associated with throat or other infections, and the following case illustrates the possibillity of Lac Caninum being useful in this condition. A man of 43 complained of a left-sided sore throat. Empty swallowing or swallowing liquids was more painful than eating solids. The tongue was heavily coated and the breath very offensive. There were stabs of pain shooting into the ear. The symptoms shifted to the right side and then back to the left. Lac Caninum was given and a very rapid recovery was made. This man had had acute nephritis six months previously.

Mammary Glands and Lactation
It is well known that drugs may have a special affinity for a certain region of the body for no apparent reason. It may be a coincidence, but there is a hint that certain substances in potency have an affinity for the locality in which they are concentrated in a crude form in the body. For example, Calc. Carb., Phosphorus and Calc. Phos. are often used in diseases of the bone such as rickets. It is known also that Cholesterinum in potency has apparently a selective action on the liver and gallbladder. Cholecystitis may be associated with angina pectoris and Cholesterinum has a surprising effect on some of these cases.

Either for that reason or for its endocrine effect, Lac Caninum markedly affects the mammary glands. A well established feature is engorgement, fullness and pain before menstruation, worse for any jarring. There is sufficient evidence clinically also to say that Lac Caninum has almost a specific effect on the discomfort of the breasts during weaning. In fact, so marked is the effect of Lac Caninum in this direction that most people hesitate to prescribe it during lactation unless weaning is intended. It is understandable that in the interests of the mother's economy the drain of lactation might have to be stopped, and that the correctly-chosen remedy might have this effect. Lac Caninum has been used with great success in acute mastitis in nursing mothers. In fact, it is almost considered specific for this. It is probable that we are unduly concerned with the danger of the mother losing her milk. It is a different matter when weaning is desired and the powerful stimuli of sucking and emptying the breasts are absent.

A mother had difficulty in feeding her first child. The breasts were engorged but secreted very little milk and there was a considerable amount of pain. She decided not to breast-feed her second child and was given stilboestrol while in hospital. The result was not satisfactory, and eight days after the child was born she had engorged painful breasts. Lac Caninum 200c was given two-hourly and next day there was a considerable improvement. The remedy was given four-hourly and on the third day the breasts were practically normal. Ten days later the right breast became hard and secreted some milk. Lac Caninum 200c was given at two-hourly intervals. This was followed rapidly by relief of symptoms and no further trouble occurred. It may be that stilboestrol was not properly given, but the point is not essentially a comparison of the two methods, but to show that Lac Caninum apparently had some effect on lactation. It appears to influence even carcinoma of the breast.

Menstruation and Pregnancy
Lac Caninum has an effect on menstruation. The flow may be profuse or very scanty, and the menstrual period may be too soon. It has a clinical record in dysmenorrhea, and in complaints of pregnancy in anxious, restless, sensitive mothers. It will be remembered that considerable pain and fullness may occur in the breasts before the period, and a sore throat may accompany the flow. There may be constipation before and after menstruation. It can produce a strongly marked bearing-down sensation, as in Lilium Tigrinum.

Alimentary System
In the alimentary system, the appetite may be increased. There is often a craving for milk, less often an aversion to milk, and rarely an allergic sensitivity to milk. It is the one remedy with a desire for pepper, which may be combined with a desire for other condiments. The case described of rheumatism following a streptococcal throat infection had the opposite – a dislike for mustard. Lac Caninum is a remedy of opposites.

A woman who had as a child been allergic to milk complained of a curious symptom – of pain in her veins which became more prominent in little knots here and there over the surface of the trunk and limbs. The veins in one area subsided, and then another place would become involved in an irregular manner. The veins stood out and became painful in an area of about two square inches at a time. She described her menstrual periods as consisting of 'a few practically dry clots'. Lac Caninum was followed by relief from the painful veins and the next menstruation was normal for the first time in years.

Lac Caninum is to be thought of for ulceration in the mouth. The milky white coating of the tongue or inner surface of the cheek may be present, or the mucous membrane may have the glazed appearance. Alternation of sides again may draw attention to it. One peculiar sensation is that of fullness in the pelvis, or in the uterus, as if it might burst. Urging to stool with or without constipation affected most of the provers.

Micturition

There is frequency of urination, sometimes dysuria, or pain if micturition is delayed. It is stated to be a specific in enuresis. This is, of course, not true. In dealing with that difficult problem the homoeopathic part of the treatment, and I believe it is only part of the treatment, is to give the constitutional remedy, which in many cases is not apparently related to micturition. For example, in the outpatients' department we had a child who appeared to be cured by Pneumococcin 10M.

Summary

Lac Caninum is a remedy of wide application. Its mental states, such as forgetfulness, mental depression, anxiety, restlessness and sensitivity, and its fear of various sorts, are almost as strongly marked as the better-known visions or dreams of snakes. Its action on the throat has been emphasised – the appearance of the throat may give an early clue to its use. Conditions such as acute rheumatism and acute nephritis, which have throat infection as part of their pathological picture, are potential fields for the use of this and other throat remedies. The action of Lac Caninum on the mammary glands has been stressed, for painful breasts before menstruation, for acute mastitis and during the weaning period. It is a remedy for ulceration of the mouth. It has urinary symptoms but is not a specific for enuresis. It has many kinds of pain, but sharp twinges or darting pains are characteristic. It is a remedy of opposites. Irregularly shifting symptoms are almost as commonly found as alternation from side to side.

Chapter 21

Osteoarthritic Nosode

There are a number of clinical types of osteoarthritis, including that of the hips in elderly males, menopausal arthritis of knees, arthritis at various levels of the spine and generalised osteoarthritis. Despite the attitude that osteoarthritis is not a constitutional disease, constitutional homoeopathic treatment may be extremely effective.

It has been fully demonstrated in osteoarthritis of the hip that a high osteotomy of the femur may be followed by regeneration of articular cartilage, and in some instances even by development of a radiologically normal head of femur and restored joint function. This has been the favourite conservative operation in the UK for a generation. It should then be possible to achieve regeneration in any joint. In my experience the hip joint has been the most difficult to influence satisfactorily by homoeopathy, but many have been in a very advanced pathological state, and in patients unwilling to diet. Even the loss of some pounds may make a distinct difference.

Osteoarthritis of the spine usually responds to manipulation plus homoeopathy. The manipulations must, however, be done gently, simply freeing the joints with the very minimum of pain, and never in the acute stage. In osteoarthritis of hands and feet manipulation has a place, as in fact in any joint. In cases of osteoarthritis of the hands and feet, whether localised there or when it it is a part of a generalised disease, or especially when there is an admixture of rheumatoid arthritis with it, two pathological remedies have proved satisfactory in the majority of cases thus treated. This treatment consists of giving Hecla Lava 6c in alternation with Manganum 6c, twelve, twenty-four or forty-eight hours apart according to severity of symptoms for about a month, then spreading out the doses according to the degree of improvement for another month or two.

A woman of 72 suffered from a combination of osteoarthritis of the hands and feet and of rheumatoid arthritis. She was overweight and could scarcely walk. This treatment cleared it up in about three months and she remained well for over two years, when there was a slight relapse. Again this treatment cleared it up quite quickly.

There is no reason why one should not combine this treatment with occasional higher potencies of individually indicated medicines. It was suggested to me that synovial fluid or one of its constituents might be a causal factor, or a factor in perpetuating the disease once it had commenced. Potencies were made from synovial fluid taken from an osteoarthritic knee – the joint most commonly affected of all – with the object of finding out whether it might influence the disease beneficially when given in the potentised form. In an attempt to gain maximal experience of the nosode, samples were sent to several homoeopathic doctors in the UK and elsewhere. A number of these physicians have expressed their opinion that it is a valuable remedy. So far reports have indicated that the Osteoarthritic nosode is valuable in cases which have been treated constitutionally and have benefited, but which have come to a standstill. For example, I have had one such report in respect of osteoarthritis of the knee joints helped by Medorrhinum. I have also had the same experience with Sepia and other remedies. In all these cases three doses of the nosode 30c given four hours apart produced a dramatic result.

I have also used the nosode intercurrently with constitutional medicines, and tentatively as a carrier with such remedies as Ruta and Rhus Tox., mainly in acute exacerbations when the Osteoarthritic nosode 30c, combined, say, with Ruta can be given four or six hourly for some days. Obviously one cannot obtain accurate indications for its use in this way. The Osteoarthritic nosode seems to affect all joints, including those of the spine. I have had the most consistently good results with it in menopausal or post-menopausal arthritis of the knee joints, given intercurrently with individually indicated remedies.

So far, all one can say is that the Osteoarthritic nosode is a useful adjunct in the homoeopathic treatment of osteoarthritis, but the indications have not as yet been established. A proving would be worthwhile, as there is already ample encouragement to test this remedy clinically.

Chapter 22

Pyrogen

The word pyrogen, literally meaning 'fire producer', is now generally accepted to mean substances derived from bacteria, moulds, viruses, white blood corpuscles or damaged tissue cells capable of causing fever. It has been established that the most powerful pyrogens are lipopolysaccharides, which are especially to be found in the endotoxins of gram-negative bacteria.

Potentised Pyrogen
Following experiments made on animals by Dr Burden Sanderson in 1875, Dr Drysdale, realising the potential of such substances in homoeopathic practice, made a similar preparation by exposing lean beef in water to the sun's rays for three weeks. After sterilising the offensive mass he potentised it to 6c, from which much of the early work was done. Later Swan ran it up to the CM, and the American work was done mainly with the higher potencies. In the animal experiments the following signs and symptoms were found, and much as one may dislike such experiments, they form a basis on which to recall the remedy picture of Pyrogen as used in homoeopathy. The animals rapidly developed fever, with shivering, restlessness, thirst and vomiting, offensive diarrhoea with mucous and later bloody stools. When death occurred it was from heart failure.

The Remedy Picture of Pyrogen Fever
Temperature rising rapidly, intense heat, dislike of uncovering, fever with chilliness, chill begins between scapulae. Excessive sweating without relief. Coldness and chilliness that no fire can warm, general coldness of bones and extremities. It is in bold type in Dr Gibson Miller's 'cold' remedies. In addition to these symptoms fairly comparable to those derived from animal experiments, we have evidence from generations of homoeopathic practice. These include face and ears red as if blood would burst through.

Sometimes Pyrogen has to be differentiated from Belladonna and other remedies when there is hot dry skin, the heat of which remains on the examiner's hands some time afterwards. The following remedies have this symptom – Belladonna, Ferrum Phos., Veratrum Viride, Baptisia, Stramonium, Pulsatilla, Sulphur, Psorinum and Lycopodium. It is not very often found in Pyrogen although it does occur.

Swan went so far as to declare that Pyrogen was indicated in all cases when the onset of fever was accompanied with pain in the limbs. Urging to urinate at the onset of fever is another feature of Pyrogen. Delirium characterised by the sensation of being crowded with arms and legs is not uncommon; or disorientation regarding the position of his body like Baptisia, from which it may be difficult to distinguish. It is said that if temperature is very high in such circumstances, Pyrogen should be given. Palpitation is a feature of Pyrogen which is not infrequently a pointer. As the older writers put it, 'Consciousness of the heart's action'. Throbbing of the blood vessels of the neck.

Restlessness
This is a well-known symptom of Pyrogen and a pointer to its consideration in any fever. Rhus Tox. has compulsion to move; there is an aggravation from initial movement and relief from subsequent movement. Pyrogen has to keep moving. Dr Tyler described an epidemic of influenza for which Pyrogen was the main remedy. As she put it, 'One remembers the agony of restlessness with the utter impossibility of remaining for more than one moment in any position, till from a chair one wriggled and twisted in search of relief, till down on the floor, when one had to start again.' There are many restless remedies, but Arsenicum Alb. is a common one in acute conditions. Here the restlessness is mental, often accompanied by fear of death, especially around midnight. The Arsenicum patient may actually move from one bed to another.

Thirst, Vomiting and Diarrhoea
Pyrogen is in black type in Kent's *Repertory* under 'Extreme thirst'. Pyrogen shares with Phosphorus a peculiar symptom 'Vomiting of water when it becomes warm in the stomach'. Burnett wrote a pamphlet on Pyrogen in the treatment of typhoid fever. During the war while serving in India, I found Pyrogen and Arsenicum Alb. the most commonly indicated remedies in outbreaks of dysentery. In any case of vomiting and diarrhoea, without other information, I first think of these two remedies. Offensive stools are characteristic of Pyrogen; Boericke says: 'diarrhoea horribly offensive, brown-black, painless, involuntary', It also

has constipation, with complete inertia (Opium), obstinate from impaction, stools large, black and carrion-like, or small black balls (Opium).

Offensiveness

Not only may there be offensive stools. Pyrogen has offensiveness from all parts of the body including breath, menses, lochia, and occasionally sputum or urine. It has offensive pus from abscesses, including varicose ulcers which surprisingly can sometimes respond to homoeopathic treatment without other methods of dealing with impaired nutrition due to venous congestion.

Pyrogen has an extensive record in successfully dealing with puerperal sepsis. H. C. Allen recommended Pyrogen for septic fevers, especially puerperal. Kent says that Pyrogen 'when indicated, can cure puerperal sepsis in a few hours'. It has offensive lochia, suppressed lochia, lochia suppressed from getting chilled. Pyrogen has been found useful in dealing with retained placenta. H. C. Allen suggested that the administration of Pyrogen acted by raising the vital activity of the uterus, thus enabling it to expel its contents. Both Pyrogen and Pulsatilla have been claimed to be effective in retained placenta in cattle. Another well-tested use of Pyrogen is in chronic ill-health after abortion or a severe labour, even without any obvious pelvic pathology, and in the absence of offensive odours or any other symptoms of Pyrogen. In uterine bleeding, when the blood is bright red and the patient has a clean tongue accompanied by nausea, Ipecacuanha is indicated, but if there is no response Pyrogen may be effective. Pyrogen often has a dirty tongue, with brown fur or a brown streak. It has cured cases of blood poisoning and is also sometimes useful when ill health dates from dental extraction.

Nephritis

Clarke quotes a case of nephritis treated by Pyrogen which deserves careful consideration. A woman aged fifty had been under treatment for Bright's disease at various hospitals, including the Hahnemann Hospital in New York, to which she was re-admitted in March 1890 under the care of Dr Dillingham. The urine showed an enormous amount of albumin and a variety of casts. Feet and legs greatly swollen, face puffy. Throbbing headache, often accompanied by nosebleed, nausea and vomiting, worse for motion and light; abnormally bright eyes, widely dilated pupils. Belladonna gave temporary relief, but the condition soon became desperate. Dr Dillingham then learned that the trouble dated from a large abscess resulting from a lanced, badly managed felon of the left thumb. She was ill six weeks with this abscess, having, as her doctor said, 'blood poisoning'. Soon after this her face and feet began to swell. On the 31st May the condition was this: feet, legs and genitals greatly swollen, frightful throbbing headache better for tight band constantly worn, or heat, very fond of hot baths. Headaches had terrible aggravations lasting two to four days, during which time she could neither lie in bed nor sit up, but was in constant motion, groaning and crying piteously for help. One dose of Pyrogen CM was given, and although the patient on one occasion begged for something to relieve the pain nothing else was given. In the course of June she began to mend and on the 20th October she was discharged cured.

Heart Failure
One of the most definite pointers to Pyrogen is a relative tachycardia in fever, which may, as already stated, be accompanied by palpitation. Occasionally there is a relatively slower pulse, possibly caused by heart block. Pyrogen was said to be effective in some epidemics of diphtheria, as might be expected with its typical myocarditis.

Bronchopneumonia
A boy of 18 months was admitted to the children's ward in the morning, having developed the first symptoms of bronchopneumonia during the previous evening. I put him on Lycopodium 200c two-hourly, but when I saw him that evening there was no improvement in his condition. In these circumstances there is almost always some sign of improvement in eight or ten hours at the most, with the right remedy. A routine throat swab taken on admission showed the presence of Vincent's angina. There were no obvious symptoms pointing to another remedy, and I considered prescribing penicillin as he was quite ill. The chart showed a marked discrepancy between pulse and temperature with a relative tachycardia, and I put him on Pyrogen 200c two-hourly, but asked the night sister to call me if there was any change for the worse, and to give him penicillin immediately. He was much better in the morning and a throat swab demonstrated that the Vincent's angina had disappeared. He had not needed penicillin. He made an uneventful recovery but was rather slow in finally clearing up. He was given Psorinum, which is complementary to Pyrogen, with apparently good results. In this case there were no other symptoms such as restlessness, offensiveness, etc.

Subsequently I have prescribed Pyrogen on the basis of relative tachycardia, or a swinging temperature when a septic focus was present, when apparently indicated remedies failed, often in the absence of any other Pyrogen symptoms and almost always successfully.

Pyrogen has proved useful in the treatment of influenza, especially in the later stages when a relative tachycardia was present.

Dr Tyler quoted a number of interesting cases treated by Pyrogen reported by a Dr Sherbino, who referred to Pyrogen as 'this great nosode . . . one of the greatest monuments to Hahnemann and to homoeopathy, as it covers a very wide range of action and fills a place of its own that no other can fill.'

OTHER PYROGENS

Swan potentised 'the contents of a septic abscess' and called it Septicaeminum, which from its origin is obviously another Pyrogen. The only information I can find is as follows: A supply was given to a soldier fighting in the South African war, with instructions to take a globule every four hours if attacked by anything like sinking or typhoid fever. The young man wrote home that 'Septicaeminum is like magic in diarrhoea and dysentery in camp life', and asked for more as his supply was largely drawn on by his friends.

Shortly after World War Two we admitted a number of patients into the Royal London Homoeopathic Hospital suffering from osteomyelitis, children who had received antibiotic treatment with sterile pus still flowing. They all cleared up on homoeopathic treatment with inter-current doses of individual 30c potencies of their pus. It has long been customary in homoeopathic practice to consider potentised pus as a remedy when the discharge is profuse and chronic. Long before chemo-therapy came to the rescue, homoeopathic treatment with individually selected remedies was claimed to cure some cases of osteomyelitis, providing sequestrae were removed, and this I can confirm from experience.

Chapter 23

Sol

Considering the already unwieldy materia medica, a vast extension would be of doubtful value. However, much more attention should be given to the choice of new remedies to be proved. All life on earth depends upon the sun's rays, but at the same time these can be dangerous, for example causing skin cancer, and their effect can be lethal, as for example in cases of severe sunstroke.

Sol is prepared by exposing saccharum lactis to concentrated sun's rays, 'stirred with a glass rod till saturated'. Potencies are then made in the usual way. A chapter on Sol is to be found in Clarke's *Dictionary of the Materia Medica*.

I was treating a man suffering from sun dermatitis, which he had developed in Egypt during the war. Non-homoeopathic treatment had failed to produce results, and after comparative failure to relieve the condition by apparently indicated homoeopathic remedies I prescribed Sol 1M, and the skin rapidly cleared up. During the following three years he had three relapses, cleared up each time on a prescription of Sol 1M, one dose. He had no trouble during the next four years, after which I lost touch with him.

An Italian woman of twenty-six years suffered from sun dermatitis, for which she had been given Pulsatilla 200c by an Italian doctor with very good effect. When she came to live in England I repeated the Pulsatilla when the condition regressed, also with good results, but she had still to avoid exposure to sunshine for any length of time. A daily dose of Sol 30c for three days was followed by an excellent and long-lasting effect.

A man of thirty complained of hay fever, which he had suffered from for three years following sunstroke. The only definite modality I could discover was that he was invariably worse on exposure to sunshine. A dose of Sol 200c was followed by cessation of the hay fever for that summer. Hay fever returned the following year, and after a prescription of Sol it again disappeared. This happened a third time after which he had no more trouble. I have no record of the pollen count in this case, but subsequently found that a *few* patients had aggravations related to exposure to sunlight, irrespective of pollen counts, with such a history.

In the children's outpatients' department of the Royal London Homoeopathic Hospital some years ago, we kept a look out for children who were unduly sensitive to sunlight, either in the way of excess freckling and/or inability to withstand exposure to sunlight in the summer months.

A girl of eleven years of age, who freckled excessively, was being treated for cheiropompholyx. This child seemed to be typically of Phosphorus type, and Phosphorus covers eruptions between the fingers. Phosphorus in various potencies failed to produce any effect, and Carcinosin was given on the basis of family history and failure of a related remedy. Again there was no obvious response. A dose of Sol 1M was tried, after which the cheiropompholyx cleared up within a month. There was a slight relapse some months later, which rapidly subsided after a further dose of Sol 1M was given.

A boy of seven suffered from sunburn from the least exposure to sun during the summer, which is unusual in the UK. Three doses of Sol 200c, every six hours in one day was given. With reasonable precautions the boy did not burn excessively for the whole of that summer. He was given the same prescription at the beginning of each summer for the next two years, with good effect, after which I lost track of him. This prescription since then has protected a great many children and adults.

A middle-aged man, with a long history of sun dermatitis, from which his father had also suffered, was helped by Sol. At first in potencies 6c, 9c and 12c, later by 1M with other remedies. At one stage he complained of pain at the site of a skin biopsy which had been performed eighteen years previously. This area became painful and began to scale excessively. In this case there was a strong history of cancer and other symptoms suggesting Carcinosin. Previous experience led me to add Carcinosin to the list of medicines 'Wounds slow to heal', and under the circumstances it seemed appropriate to consider Carcinosin in the treatment of this patient. Carcinosin 30c was followed by a slight aggravation, then considerable general improvement.

A woman of sixty had a colostomy, along with the removal of a malignant tumour of the large intestine. She was under my care for post-operative treatment and kept reasonably well for five years following the operation. Then her general health deteriorated, although careful examination did not reveal any recurrence of the growth. Radiotherapy was then given, and following this she found that she could not stand being exposed to the least sunlight, whereas she had been a keen sunbather as far back as she could remember, including during the post-operative period. I prescribed Sol 30c daily, one dose for three days, with excellent effect. This had to be repeated some months later, and on subsequent occasions after radiotherapy, also with good effect. She died at the age of eighty.

This led me to prescribe Sol 30c routinely to counteract the adverse effects of radiotherapy, giving three doses every two hours commencing after radiation, or otherwise depending on the time of day that radiotherapy was given. Patients who had been given radiation previously claimed that the Sol treatment was highly effective.

In a case of Hodgkin's disease the experienced radiotherapist, who was unaware that Sol treatment had been given, expressed surprise at the very rapid regrowth of pubic hair following radiation of the inguinal glands.

Occasionally the onset of ill-health may be associated with extensive diagnostic X-rays. Limited experience suggested that Sol 200c was superior to X-ray 200c in such cases.

Some years ago I treated three cases of severe adverse effects of Cobalt radiation following mastectomy as follows. Sol 200c six doses every two hours on the first day, Sol 200c every three hours on the second day, and four doses every four hours on third and fourth days; then Sol 200c three doses every six hours on days five, six, and seven, keeping a careful watch to stop after full relief was secured, which was about the end of the week in all three cases. Two had a slight relapse which responded to Sol 200c three doses every twelve hours. I lost touch with two of the cases, but by chance found that the third one had had no relapse seven years later.

Chapter 24

Tarentula Hispanica

Two common symptom complexes leading to a prescription of Tarentula Hispanica are: (1) Sudden outburst of destructiveness occurring only when the child is, or thinks he is, not being observed, and (2) 'Feigning sickness'. Clinical details of the cases chosen have been omitted in order to emphasise the homoeopathic indications.

A boy of six years with rheumatic chorea appeared to be a quiet, good-natured little fellow on ward rounds, but Sister told us that he was, as she put it, 'foxy – when he thinks no one is watching him he may suddenly tear up his books and smash any toys he can lay his hands on.' Tarentula 10M was followed by a dramatic change. His bouts of destructiveness stopped and he made a rapid recovery.

A boy of eight years was admitted partly because of an atypical primary tuberculous complex, and also because he suffered from an anxiety state. There was a strong history of tuberculosis in the family and the boy had been under observation in the outpatients' department on this account. The primary complex was clearing up. He was nervous, excitable, obstinate, destructive, and very jealous of his younger sister aged six years. While in the ward it was noted that he had many complaints, which were turned on at suitable times and for which no physical cause could be found. When he thought no one was watching him he sometimes got out of bed, hit one of the other children, and then dashed into bed again. Tarentula Hispanica 30c, 200c, 1M on three consecutive days was followed by a rapid and sustained improvement in the boy's mental state.

A boy of six years is at present recovering from a fairly severe attack of rheumatic fever – his second one. Like the previous case, he was extremely obstinate and Tub. Bov. 200c seemed to help him. It had also appeared to help him in his previous attack. He was not however making very much progress, and after a conference with the ward sister, the following picture emerged. He was always wide awake after the other children were asleep and remained awake till eleven or twelve o'clock, quite bright and cheerful as a rule. He was correspondingly sleepy in the mornings. He was a pleasant and apparently placid child, but at times when he became annoyed he would have a bout of destructiveness – tearing up books and breaking toys. He would hit out at nurses with whom he was usually extremely friendly. Until restraint was put on him, there was considerable difficulty in keeping him in bed, even when he was quite ill. He would suddenly get out of bed and run around the ward wildly. Tarentula is not noted in Kent's *Repertory* under the symptom 'obstinacy', but otherwise there was a close similarity. His recovery has been rapid since a prescription of Tarentula 30c, 200c, 1M.

A girl of eight years was causing considerable parental concern on account of her inability to concentrate at school, although her IQ was well above average. This child was treated in the outpatients' department for over a year without very much benefit, until the mother confessed that there was something else which was causing even greater anxiety. The child was a kleptomaniac. She stole objects usually of little or no value and hid them. Other symptoms of Tarentula were present. Tarentula Hispanica 30c, 200c, 1M was given three months ago and her teachers have already reported progress. There have been no further stealing episodes.

Footnote. The prescription of a remedy in three ascending potencies was a favourite method of Dr Tyler's. Various sequences may be given in this way. In the case of a 30c, 200c, 1M, a single dose of 30c is given on the first day, a dose of 200c on the second and 1M on the third. It is used mainly in chronic or sub-acute conditions; it possibly gives a wider range of stimulus and is believed to minimise the risk of severe aggravation.

Chapter 25

The Constitutional Effects of Anaesthesia

It has long been recognised in homoeopathic practice that constitutional treatment may be interfered with by the after-effects of prolonged or unsuitable drugging. Generations of homoeopaths have, for instance, been able to antidote the adverse influence of prolonged taking of quinine by Natrum Mur., Natrum Sulph. and other remedies according to individual requirements. Nux Vomica has a reputation for the after-effects of drugging in general and in Boericke's *Materia Medica* there is a list of remedies associated with 'abuse of drugs'. Also, there are several references scattered through the homoeopathic literature to a method of antidoting after-effects of drugs to which a patient is unduly sensitive by administering the offending drug in potency. For example, Sulphapyridine was found useful in this respect shortly after the introduction of the sulphonamide group of drugs, and it is sometimes possible by this method to antidote the after-effects of many of the modern powerful drugs. For reasons not at present clear, the administration of a drug in potency to antidote its after-effects may or may not be successful.

Among the drugs widely prescribed today are those acting as depressants of the central nervous system, including anaesthetics, hypnotics and narcotics, all having an action in common in lessening consciousness. While there are occasional references to antidoting one of the hypnotics or narcotics, the anaesthetic drugs have been almost completely neglected. This whole group of drugs are well worth studying.

A routine enquiry into the anaesthetic history of patients during the past year and attempts to antidote by giving the anaesthetic drug in potency has been rewarding. Modern anaesthesia is complex and it may be impossible to find out which of the drugs employed is at fault. Not infrequently, however, there is a clear-cut history of patients being unduly upset by chloroform, ether or nitrous oxide. The most definite picture which has emerged from this study is that of chloroform, an account of which is to be found in Clark's *Dictionary*, Hering's *Guiding Symptoms* and elsewhere in the homoeopathic materia medica. For patients unduly upset by chloroform, who give a history of hepatic disorder or gallbladder disease, Chloroform 30c may be a valuable remedy.

Case 1. A woman of 70 complained of recurrent bouts of flatulent dyspepsia associated with discomfort under the right scapula. At the age of 67 she had been operated on for gallstones which were removed, but not the gallbladder. After a stormy post-operative period complicated by a pulmonary embolus, the patient remained weak and her flatulent attacks persisted. Chelidonium 3x and 6x was an effective remedy to relieve flatulence. Her constitutional remedy seemed to be Sepia and this was given with some benefit, but not as much as might have been expected. Enquiry into the anaesthetic history revealed that she had had six previous operations, all under chloroform, which upset her considerably; she was always violently sick afterwards. Chloroform 30c was given, which was followed by a remarkable improvement in the patient's appearance and general health and comparative freedom from attacks for six months. An interesting feature was that her perspiration, which left brown stains, became clear soon after the Chloroform was given. There was a slight relapse after six months and Chloroform 100c was given. This was followed by a 'cold' and epigastric pain for two days and then further improvement.

Case 2. A boy of 8 was seen on account of frequent attacks of bronchitis accompanied by vomiting. There was some evidence of infection of the tonsils and adenoids and the boy lost weight after an attack; this was rapidly regained, and was probably not associated with sepsis in the upper respiratory tract. The constitutional remedy appeared to be Carcinosin, which he was given in the 30c, 200c and 1M potency on three consecutive days. Apart from sleeping better, the results were unsatisfactory. The remedy seemed clearly indicated, but in view of the poor response the history was re-examined. The only outstanding event in his personal history was an operation for pyloric stenosis. Two tablets of Chloroform 30c were given and placebo was sent on. A month later his mother reported: 'On the way home after we saw you last month Michael developed a colicky pain in his tummy. It returned two days later and again on the fourth day, when it was so bad he was sent home from school. Since then he has been very much better in every way and the pain has not returned. Also, he has had much less trouble with his school work.' This case illustrates two important aspects of antidoting anaesthesia. Firstly, there may be an abreactive effect, as it were, a 'lifting of unconsciousness'.

Secondly, the 'lifting of unconsciousness' may be followed by increased alertness. In the case of any child who is reported from school to be intelligent but not using his brain, it is worthwhile to consider one of the anaesthetics or other drugs of the central nervous system depressant group according to the history. Nitrous oxide should not be dismissed in this respect on theoretical grounds.

Case 3. A woman of 42 had been treated for chronic nasal catarrh, mainly by Sepia and with considerable success. She had fractured her femur at the age of 25 and, owing to mismanagement, had spent some years of misery. Osteoarthritis of the left hip joint was well established. In September Chloroform 30c was given. The following January, when she was next seen, she reported: 'I have been very much better generally and this is the first time in my life I have been able to face my operation.'

Case 4. A mentally backward child had been treated at the Royal London Homoeopathic Hospital for four years with some benefit. Enquiry into the anaesthetic history revealed that the mother had a 'whiff of gas' at his birth. Nitrous Oxide 30c was given experimentally and two months later the mother reported: 'Within a week after beginning the last course of treatment Ian became much more alert.'

Case 5. A woman of 20 complained of bouts of colicky epigastric pains which began at the age of 8. The attacks had become much more frequent and more severe during the previous year. Investigations were all negative. Colocynth 3x was found to be an effective remedy in relieving the pains, but despite careful constitutional treatment the number of attacks, about one in two weeks, was not reduced. There was a strong family history of cancer, and four siblings had been helped by Carcinosin. Carcinosin Adeno. Stom. 30c was given, but without apparent effect. She was the only one of the family born under chloroform anaesthesia and on this fact, together with symptoms of liver dysfunction, Chloroform 30c was tried. The attacks cleared for three months and then returned, but not so severely. Chloroform 100c was given and followed by another four months' freedom except for one attack.

Case 6. A woman of 48 complained of attacks of giddiness of ten years' duration. The vertigo was so severe she was getting afraid to go out shopping. Lying down relieved the giddiness in about half a minute. She also suffered from migraine. Similar attacks had occurred for a year or two at puberty. There was no definite evidence of Menières's syndrome. The patient was intolerant of fats and eggs. Hepatic dysfunction had been diagnosed at the age of 34.

Previous Illnesses. Tonsils and adenoids removed in childhood. First labour difficult. Chloroform given, no apparent adverse after-effects. Appendicectomy performed during the second pregnancy when she was twenty-eight.

Family History. Tendency to migraine.

Clinical examination was negative except for emaciation. Blood pressure was 140/80 and there was no evidence of anaemia. The following constitutional symptoms were repertorised:

Sympathetic to others.
> Massage.
Faintness in a crowd.
Timidity – bashful.
< Cold.
Emaciation.
< before menses.
> open air.
Clothing on neck <
Clothing on abdomen <

A number of remedies including Lycopodium, Phosphorus, Natrum Carb., Sepia and Zincum were considered but none completely covered the case. There was nothing in the history to suggest a nosode, and taking into consideration the anaesthetic history, together with hepatic dysfunction, Chloroform 30c was tried. There was a definite improvement in her general health and freedom from attacks during the next month. Phosphorus and Dysentery Co. were subsequently given, and three months after commencing treatment she reported that she never felt so well in her life and had gained in weight for the first time for years.

Chapter 26

Glandular Fever

This disease is believed to be caused by Epstein Barr virus, and is said to be usually self-limiting with a very low mortality rate. Occasionally patients diagnosed as having had glandular fever, with or without laboratory evidence recent or remote, suffer from chronic ill-health afterwards, although Epstein Barr virus has not been found in these chronic cases. Some of these have recurrent episodes of adenitis, some with enlarged spleen and/or hepatitis. It is interesting to note that the Carcinosins seem to be effective in the treatment of these chronic cases, in view of the association of Epstein Barr virus with Burkitt's lymphoma and post-nasal malignancy.

I saw a young teacher who had been diagnosed as having had glandular fever three years previously, and who suffered from chronic ill-health and recurrent episodes of cervical adenitis. There was a family history and other indications of Carcinosin, including the presence of several moles. I prescribed Carcinosin 200c three doses every six hours in one day. I did not see the patient for another two years, as she worked abroad. She then reported that she had been in good health until fairly recently, when she had a slight recurrence of cervical adenitis. I repeated the prescription of Carcinosin 200c three doses every six hours, and two years later there was no report of any recurrence. I have treated a number of other similar cases in this way with success, as illustrated by the following examples.

A woman of twenty-three, a musician and teacher of music, had been diagnosed as having suffered from glandular fever three years previously. At the onset there was cervical adenitis and enlarged glands in the axilla and groin. Since then she had suffered from headaches, usually precipitated by anticipation, such as when she had to go on the stage, and she also had recurrent episodes of adenitis.

Family History. Father's father had cancer of the lungs. Mother's brother was a diabetic.

Mentals and Generals. Headaches from anticipation. Sensitive to music. Loved dancing, had done ballet training. Since the glandular fever she felt better at the seaside.

Treatment. Carcinosin 200c three doses every six hours was given, and repeated two months later when she had a slight recurrence. After that I heard no more from her, but a friend of hers came to me two years later, who had also suffered from the after-effects of glandular fever, and told me that this lady had been completely cured. The friend was also cured after treatment with Carcinosin 200c followed by Sepia 30c. In my experience this has been most often subsequently required, although it is obviously an individual matter.

When there is chronic hepatitis I have given Carcinosin Adeno. Stom. in the same way – three doses every six hours, and in such cases I have given Chelidonium mother tincture five drops in a little water t.i.d., p.c. for a month. Apart from glandular fever, this is also a useful procedure in the treatment of chronic hepatitis when Carcinosin is otherwise indicated. In such cases I have given Chelidonium in the way just outlined. If the tenderness extends to the left beyond the midline, Carduus Marianus given in the same way seems to have a better effect. Such courses may have to be repeated later on.

When the liver is tender as a complication of any acute illness, for example influenza, Chelidonium mother tincture given in this way, along with remedies for the acute illness, seems to be very helpful with or without other indications. In the treatment of acute glandular fever I have prescribed either Carcinosin or Carcinosin Adeno. Stom. 30c or 200c in the same way as one would in any acute condition, giving it three times a day, say for four days, then twice a day for four days, and then spreading out the dose as required. If an untreated patient goes slightly beyond the normal time, say two months, I would give three or four doses of Carcinosin Adeno. Stom. every twelve hours plus Chelidonium, unless there were indications for other remedies. Should the patient be considerably debilitated in any chronic disease – including the aftermath of glandular fever – it is advisable to proceed cautiously, as the following case history illustrates.

A woman of twenty-four had been unwell for three and a half years. She also had recurrent episodes of cervical adenitis following an attack of what had been diagnosed as glandular fever. She was generally weak, and especially got tired standing. On a few occasions she had fainted when standing in a warm close room. She had been very constipated, particularly during the previous two years, and had a low resistance to colds. She said that she had been off work for nine months on this account.

Past History. Tonsillectomy at nineteen. She had acne vulgaris, mainly white vesicles round the chin.

Family History. Both grandfathers had Parkinson's disease.

On Examination. Slim build. Very slight acne round the chin, white vesicles. Anaemic. No enlargement of spleen. Liver not enlarged or tender. Itchy eyes.

Mentals and Generals. Sympathetic to others. Apprehensive. Loves watching a thunderstorm. Enjoys travelling very much. Sensitive to music.
She was very much better for playing games and for exertion, but had been unable to do much in that way in the recent past. She was constipated, and only passed a stool about once a week. She did not eat very much, and had to strain very considerably to pass a stool of normal consistency.
She had an aversion to potatoes and loved fish. The type of constipation she had during the previous two years was associated with cooking with aluminium utensils. This, together with the aversion to potatoes, itchy eyes and a tendency to colds, all suggested sensitivity to aluminium. I advised discontinuation of aluminium utensils, including tin foil for oven dishes.

Treatment. I prescribed a preparation of iron, and three powders of Alumina 30c combined with Vitamin E 30c to be taken twelve hours apart, after discontinuing aluminium cooking utensils.
A month later there was a slight improvement in her condition, and the constipation was practically cured. I gave her Natrum Mur. 30c, 200c and 1M on consecutive days. Natrum Mur. covers faintness in a warm crowded room, sympathetic to others, weakness standing, better for exertion, desires fish, sensitive to music. When acne presents itself round the mouth or chin it is well worth considering Natrum Mur., especially if otherwise indicated, and it also covers the tendency to colds.
There was a further improvement and six weeks later I gave her a dose of Sepia 30c. Sepia is complementary to Natrum Mur. – it also covers the type of constipation (which had remained cured), and in my experience people of the Sepia type are very often sensitive to aluminium. Sepia also covers sympathetic to others, sudden weakness standing, room full of

people aggravates, and loves watching a thunderstorm. It is important to note that this symptom is covered not only by Sepia but by Carcinosin and Bellis Perennis as well. Her hair was greasy, and in my experience Sepia covers this also.

There was a further improvement after Sepia, and six weeks later I gave her Carcinosin 30c, followed by Carcinosin 200c a month later. The prescription of Carcinosin was delayed as the patient was very debilitated and might have reacted too strongly, and it seemed better to deal with aluminium sensitivity first. Five months later she was perfectly alright and went abroad. A report eighteen months later said that she had had no further relapses and was perfectly well. Early the following year she returned to England in excellent health, with her first baby.

Other important remedies which have influenced the after-effects of glandular fever are Glandular Fever Nosode 200c and Ailanthus Glandulosa 10M; I have used these occasionally if Carcinosin failed. One case which did not respond to Glandular Fever Nosode responded well to Carcinosin.

Chapter 27

Haemorrhoids

Constitutional prescribing is usually difficult owing to the large choice of potential remedies. However, the use of combined remedies has been successful in the majority of cases, even more so when combined with diet, which in some cases is essential. From Dr Tyler I learned the value of a routine course of Nux Vomica 3x before breakfast and Sulphur 3x on retiring, for a month. This was often completely successful, and the course could be repeated if there was a recurrence. Cases responding partially were dealt with by a further month of Nux Vomica and Sulphur on alternate days, and so on.

Unsatisfactory results in some cases led me to add Rhamnus Frangula, giving Nux Vomica, Sulphur, and Rhamnus Frangula 3x t.i.d. a.c. for a month. This effected further cures to the extent that I gave this prescription routinely. An ointment of Aesculus, Calendula, Hamamelis and Paeonia is useful also in all cases. Occasionally another remedy was individually required and could be added to the Nux and Sulphur mixture, with or without Rhamnus Frangula. These remedies most often were, in my experience, Aesculus, Hamamelis, Paeonia, Ratanhia or Ruta, in similar low potencies. All these remedies can cover pruritis and bleeding.

Whenever there is itching of the anus, haemorrhoids or perineum, consideration must be given to avoiding food or drink heated in aluminium vessels, and also alcohol, especially draught beer stored in aluminium containers. Eggs should not be boiled in an aluminium pan. Complete avoidance is almost impossible, but the evidence suggests that effects are accumulative. Patients can be advised of their personal aluminium symptoms, and the antidote, Alumina 30c three doses every six hours in one day, repeated when required.

Another aluminium rectal symptom often associated with haemorrhoids is constipation, characterised by weakness of rectal muscles to the extent that straining is required when passing even a soft stool. Alternatively, there can be an accumulation of hard stools resulting in considerable pain as well as weakness in defaecation. Less often there may be weakness of the oesophagus, resulting in a sensation of constriction during the passage of food. Another common symptom is itching of the eyes, especially the inner canthi.

Alumina is fully represented in Kent's *Repertory*, and information can be found in both Kent and Boericke's *Materia Medica*. Other sources are Allen's *Keynotes*, Tyler's *Drug Pictures*, Nash's *Leaders* and Guernsey's *Keynotes of the Materia Medica*.

Regarding diet, there was evidence from Africa that haemorrhoids were found in a much higher proportion of Europeans than in the native population in the same region, who used only cane sugar. This was before the more recent research showing that avoidance of sugar, including confectionery, jams and alcohol, is advisable for patients suffering from haemorrhoids. Replacing white bread by wholemeal bread, and using bran as a cereal, have been shown to be factors in the avoidance of haemorrhoids as well as in their treatment.

Homoeopathic treatment and diet is very effective in the vast majority of cases. Rest may be necessary, at least temporarily in some instances, and analgesics may be required. Operation may be necessary. A combination of Staphysagria, Aesculus and Bellis Perennis 30c can be given pre- and post-operatively.

Chapter 28

After-Effects of Head Injury

Head injury can occur occasionally before birth, and birth injury may be an important landmark when labour has been prolonged, or equally if it has been very rapid, or from the trauma of forceps. It is well known that failure to cry soon after birth, or difficulty in starting feeding or weaning, suggests consideration of head injury.

Failure to thrive may be associated with birth injury or very early head injury; for example, a boy of six caught cold very easily, never thrived properly and was markedly underweight. According to his mother he had no interest in life. He was very sensitive to noise and was afraid even when there was a high wind. He had other symptoms of Natrum Sulph. and a history of a difficult birth confirmed its choice as a remedy. He was given Natrum Sulph. 30c, 200c and 1M on consecutive days and this was followed by a rapid improvement in health, mentally and physically. After some months there was a slight relapse which responded very well to a repeat of the course of treatment.

Injury occurring in sport, especially rugger or boxing, car accidents, operations on sinuses or mastoidectomy, may also cause clinically significant after-effects.

A history of head injury is sometimes very difficult to obtain, but it can be of great importance in constitutional prescribing. It has long been established that there is no sharp dividing line between the post-concussion syndrome and other after-effects, which is not reflected in our repertories. The rubrics in Kent's *Repertory* 'Injury to the head, after', 'Concussion', and 'Pain, mechanical injury, after' can thus be combined, giving rise to a large general rubric, to which can be added Agaricus, Alumina, Aurum Met., Bellis Perennis, Carcinosin, Glonoin and Veratrum Alb.

Dr Royal Hayes pointed out the value of Helleborus Niger in an excellent paper published in the *Homoeopathic Recorder* of December 1948. Over several years I have found Helleborus to be a most commonly indicated remedy, and have usually prescribed it 30c, 200c and 1M on consecutive days. When there were strong partial indications for Helleborus and another remedy, the two can be combined, and I have usually prescribed the mixture also 30c, 200c and 1M on consecutive days. An outstanding symptom of Helleborus is great weakness of memory for recent events. Reporting on a prover, Hahnemann said that it was only after an effort, and after some time, that he could remember what he wanted to say and what he had been questioned about. Reporting on another he said that the person could not remember what he had read for one instant. Forgetfulness for recent events is common in old age and Helleborus does not cure it, but in younger age groups it can be worth consideration. The same applies to other remedies useful in the after-effects of head injury, but to a lesser extent.

Mental illness may be associated with head injury. The tendency for professional boxers to develop a recognised pathological pattern associated with characteristic mental changes is well known. Early this century Dr Talcott, Professor of Mental Diseases at the New York Medical Center and Homeopathic Hospital, said that in his opinion mental disease could result from head injury even several years previously. Subsequent research in the UK based on post-mortem evidence suggested a possible link between head injury and schizophrenia. Recent research carried out at the University of Helsinki provides evidence of a considerable higher incidence of morphological signs and brain dysfunction in expert boxers, both amateur and professional, compared with controls. This report is to be found in a paper entitled 'Is Chronic Brain Damage in Boxing a Hazard of the Past?', to be found in *The Lancet*, 27th December 1982.

Regarding Veratrum Alb., Hahnemann claimed that it could, along with other remedies, cure a third of the insane in a lunatic asylum (see Tyler's *Drug Pictures*). Veratrum Alb. is noted in Barthel's *Repertory* as a remedy for concussion, and as such should be taken into consideration with the other remedies when there is a history of head injury in the past.

Glonoin has a reputation for dealing effectively with the immediate after-effects of a fractured skull, and according to Tyler eliminates the need for morphine. Limited personal experience has confirmed this. In chronic conditions with such a history, Glonoin should be taken into consideration with the other head injury remedies, especially if there has been an adverse reaction to sun, such as sunstroke.

Some people report severe reaction to general anaesthesia. Limited experience suggests this may be associated with previous mechanical trauma. Potencies of the anaesthetic used have in some cases been effective, for example in children unable to study after an operation. In others, head injury remedies have been followed by improvement. My impression is that after severe head injury there is a tendency to limitation of movement of the cervical and upper dorsal vertebrae. I have in such cases given gentle manipulative treatment with the aim of normalising cerebral blood flow, and have reviewed the situation at each consultation. Whatever current views may be held, this procedure, done gently and expertly, seems to be helpful in the treatment of migraine, Menière's syndrome and mental disease. There is, however, considerable evidence that these conditions can sometimes be effectively dealt with by homoeopathy alone and without manipulation.

Another factor requiring consideration in dealing with the aftermath of head injury is that some people can be adversely affected in various ways by food or drink heated in aluminium utensils. Provings and clinical experience, recorded for example in Kent's *Repertory*, demonstrate that a wide variety of head symptoms can be caused by aluminium. Aluminium can be an allergen, and clinical experience suggests that strict avoidance of it, at least in the home, can reduce the reaction to other allergens, which may also be useful in the treatment of migraine. Dr Tyler was well aware of the effect of aluminium in sensitive subjects, and has a useful chapter on the subject in her *Homoeopathic Drug Pictures*.

Allergic Rhinitis

A young man aged 17. Profuse lacrimation and clear watery, bland, nasal discharge alternating with blocked nose. Much sneezing in the morning after rising. Said to be allergic to feathers and house dust; worse in the early summer and when the pollen count is raised. He had had this for about four years and it was getting progressively worse each year.

Another major problem was that he had great difficulty in concentrating, and although apparently intelligent, he had great difficulty in his school work and in passing examinations.

Past History. Forceps at birth. Tonsils and adenoids were operated on and a second operation was performed, as the adenoids apparently had not been successfully dealt with. He had a washing out of sinuses between the age of four and five. Puberty was delayed in comparison with a sibling, but after that he developed rapidly and became a keen and capable rugby player. He had concussion at fifteen years.

On Examination. Generally fit. No deviation of nasal septum. His mother said that he slept with his head dorsiflexed, and that he tended to snore at nights.

Mentally he was sympathetic to others, very considerate, and his

163

mother described him as a day-dreamer. He was absent-minded and forgetful of very recent events. He used to cry a lot as a young boy and was bullied, but this soon changed after puberty. Very fond of milk. He drank at least a pint a day and was also very fond of cheese.

Consideration of Treatment. It is possible that early head injuries resulted in diminished pituitary function and delayed puberty, and the more recent concussion might have caused his snoring. There was limitation of movement of the cervical vertebrae. Helleborus covers the effects of head injury, sympathetic to others, day-dreaming, loss of memory for recent events (greatly outside the norm for his age), concentration difficult, and sneezing in the morning. Natrum Mur. covers head injury, concentration difficult, sympathetic, day-dreaming, better for exertion, profuse watery nasal discharge alternating with blocked nose and sneezing.

Treatment. I advised reducing milk to not more than half a pint a day, and to avoid cheese. Gentle manipulation resulted in freeing the cervical rotation, and I prescribed Helleborus combined with Natrum Mur. 9c, 12c, and 30c on consecutive days. This was followed by freedom from snoring and general all-round improvement, which was progressive.

Two months later he had a slight injury to the neck. I freed the neck and repeated the prescription. Two months after that the report was that he was very much better generally and academically, and the allergic rhinitis was reported to be cured.

Amenorrhoea

A woman of thirty suffered from amenorrhoea since the age of eighteen, following anorexia nervosa from which she recovered sufficiently to carry on working. For some months before her first consultation she had suffered from a very painful nose, worse inspiring and worse in warmth.

On Examination. Slimly built. Nose extremely red externally and internally, no deflection of the septum and no enlargement of the cervical lymph glands.

Past History. Upbringing strict. Parents persuaded her to think that she wanted to behave according to their wishes, something she still resents. Recurrent tonsilitis, tonsils removed at four. Head injury at six, fell on the right side causing a black eye and haemorrhage from the right nostril. Cervical glands on the right side remained enlarged for some years afterwards. Menstruation started at thirteen and a half years, and after some very heavy periods at the age of eighteen the anorexia nervosa was diagnosed.

Mentals and Generals. Very depressed, and a strong sense of injustice, partly on account of being still slimly built. Avoided company. Was weepy, consolation aggravated her. Sympathetic to others. Decisions difficult. Life not worth living. Sensitive to music.

Treatment. Staphysagria 30c given on account of grief, head injury, loathing of life, amenorrhoea, weepy, consolation aggravates, and followed a week later by a low potency mixture of the following remedies, Kali. Bich., Kali Carb., and China 2x, in an attempt to deal with the nasal condition. A month later the nasal condition had improved slightly.

Graphites 30c, 200c, 1M on consecutive days was prescribed, covering amenorrhoea, decisions difficult, grief, sensitive to music, sympathetic, timidity, pain inside nose a strongly-marked symptom, and red nose. A month later there was further improvement of the nose, but still amenorrhoea. In view of the failure of apparently well-indicated remedies, I decided to prescribe a mixture on the following basis:
1) Baryta Carb. Head injury can affect pituitary function, and it covers also timidity, grief, shyness, amenorrhoea and red nose.
2) Vitamin E. On account of its known influence on the female genitalia, for example, in the the treatment of infertility.
3) Thiosinaminum. On the chance that scar tissue might have some effect on the amenorrhoea.

The following prescription was sent: Baryta Carb. 12x, Vitamin E 12x, Thiosinaminum 12x. Night and morning for a week, then one dose daily for two weeks. No further treatment was given.

Ten months later she reported that her periods had returned four months after the prescription, at first very scantily, then more normal. I gave her a copy of the prescription to be taken should there be a relapse, and have not seen her since. Despite the use of mixtures, I believe it is worthwhile to report this case, as it might add to other knowledge of the aftermath of anorexia nervosa.

Angioedema
A nursing sister of thirty complained of angioedema of five years duration, commencing after depression and insecurity on leaving home to work in a distant part of the country. The attacks started in the epigastrium with pain which extended upwards to the throat, and the oedema

was associated with swelling of the tongue and eyelids along with generalised urticaria. Plums, peaches or apricots could bring on an attack although the effects were erratic. She also suffered from dermographia.

Past History. Birth was long and difficult. She had a dog bite at the age of seven which she did not report to anyone at the time. She had another head injury at eight. She suffered from bed-wetting till she was thirteen. She said her upbringing was strict but not severe. She was top of her class until puberty, after which she could not study easily.

Family History. On the mother's side a number of relatives died of tuberculosis in childhood. Her mother's brother and her father's sister both had cancer.

On Examination. Slightly overweight. Some restriction of cervical and upper dorsal spinal movement, other N.A.D.

Mentals and Generals. She was shy, made few friends but enjoyed her own company, especially in the evenings. Memory for immediate past was very poor for her age. Sensitive to music. Sympathetic and loved sympathy. She was startled easily from noise. Very chilly hands and feet. She had an intense dislike of warm drinks, and had to put much milk in her tea to cool it down.

Consideration of Treatment. Repertorisation showed indications for Arsenicum Alb., Calc. Phos., Conium, Lachesis, Phosphorus and Pulsatilla, all related to Carcinosin and the after-effects of head injury. Together with the family history this led to the prescription of Carcinosin 200c, one dose, after manipulation of the cervical and upper dorsal spine. This resulted in some improvement, although not very much.

Reassessment on the basis of head injury, the onset associated with emotional insecurity, her sensitivity to cold, especially hands and feet, aversion to warm drinks, with her memory symptoms so common after head injury, led to prescription of Helleborus 30c, 200c, 1M on consecutive days. This led to a considerable improvement, and her antihistamine could be cut down from four to two tablets daily.

This improvement, however, did not seem to be progressive. Opium 1M was given on account of its usefulness in after-effects of head injury, besides the possibility that the fright she had on being bitten by a dog, an incident which she did not report, might have had a lasting effect. There seemed to be some improvement, but the situation was unsatisfactory.

In view of the definite improvement after Helleborus, I prescribed Helleborus 1M combined with Thyroidinum 1M, one dose, on account of its effect on allergic conditions. This was followed by some improvement, although the situation was still not satisfactory. The next prescription was Conium 30c, 200c, 1M on consecutive days on account of her inability to study after puberty. Conium is a head injury remedy also and covers other aspects. This again was not fully satisfactory.

Carcinosin was then reconsidered on the original basis plus the possibility that it could cover the stress of puberty. Carcinosin 30c combined with Thyroidinum 30c, three doses every four hours in one day, was given six months from the beginning of her treatment. This was followed by a marked general improvement, the dermographia ceased and she had very occasional attacks without urticaria. This was followed one month later by Pulsatilla 30c, 200c, 1M on consecutive days, and she reported no further attacks.

I did not see her again until a further five months afterwards, when she complained of gross obesity resulting from a ravenous appetite without relish. Helleborus also covers this, and she was given Helleborus 30c, 200c, 1M on consecutive days. It dealt with the obesity problem and two years later she stated that she had continued to be perfectly well.

Footnote: I am indebted to Dr S. K. Ghosh of Calcutta for his book *Clinical Experience With Some Rare Nosodes* (1956), which includes Thyrodinum and other sarcodes. I have found that Thyroidinum can be combined, as in this case, with individually selected constitutional remedies in allergic diseases.

Anorexia Nervosa

A girl of thirteen. Five months before I first saw her she had been in hospital, where she had had a manipulation of her left knee joint, followed ten days later by removal of the cartilage. She had been very sick after both anaesthetics, and following the removal of the cartilage was in extreme pain, which did not respond to analgesics. She came home very depressed and since then her appetite had been very poor, resulting in considerable loss of weight. She looked like a slim ten-year old. Mentally she was in an apathetic stage, and had talked of suicide. Previously she had been an affectionate, responsive child, but had lately lost all interest in the family.

Past History. Concussion twice at the age of three or four. Measles badly at seven and tonsillectomy at nine, after which she was sick from the anaesthetic.

Family History. Mother's mother and grandmother died of cancer. Father's sister and aunt suffered from diabetes. There were other strong indications for Carcinosin, and also for the combined remedies Helleborus and Natrum Mur.

Treatment. I first prescribed Natrum Mur. 1M combined with Helleborus 1M, followed ten days later by Carcinosin Adeno. Stom. 30c. There was only a slight improvement. The next prescription a month later was Folliculinum 30c because of strong resentment by the patient towards her parents, as they prevented her changing to a school she very greatly preferred. There was no further improvement and talk of suicide became more prominent. I gave Aurum Met. 30c, 200c, 1M on consecutive days and she ceased to mention suicide, but her condition in general was still not satisfactory.

I went carefully over the history again and gave her Opium CM on the possibility that she had been at one time or another frightened while in hospital, and because of failure of apparently-indicated remedies. Opium covered the state of apathy and indifference to pleasure. Opium is also a remedy for the after-effects of head injury and anaesthesia. This was rapidly followed by a great improvement and three months later she returned from a skiing holiday, well and happy with a normal appetite and increased weight. No further treatment was required.

Chronic Nasal Catarrh
A boy aged twelve. Born without anaesthetic between 6 a.m. and breakfast time. Did not cry shortly after birth and was slow to start feeding. Recurrent tonsillitis and otitis media. Tonsils and adenoids removed at age seven with some improvement, but heavy catarrh continued. Pneumonia without fever.

Family History. Both parents suffered from catarrh.

On Examination. Slightly underweight. Facial oedema. No deviation of nasal septum. (When there is appreciable deviation, cure of catarrh is difficult or impossible without operation.)

Mentals. Sympathetic. Very poor memory, tends to forget what he has just read. Fastidious about clothes, otherwise untidy. (A superficial tidiness suggests consideration of Sulphur.)

Physical Generals. Lazy, 'lies about'. Loves cream and curry. Never perspires. The history of rapid birth and other indications mentioned point to head injury. The type of memory is outside the norm in a boy of twelve and suggests Helleborus Niger, alone or with a related remedy. Carcinosin was suggested by the symptoms, being partly covered by related remedies and absence of fever in pneumonia. Carcinosin is also a head injury remedy.

Treatment. Helleborus 30c, 200c, 1M was given on consecutive days, followed by Carcinosin 30c a week later, with instructions to avoid cream and restrict milk and cheese, as these foods are better avoided in such cases. He was at boarding school and a more strict regime was not practicable.

Treatment Continued. A slight improvement only was reported later, which suggested reassessment. The next prescription was Helleborus 30c, 200c, 1M, combined with Mucobacter 30c, 200c, 1M on consecutive days. (In a number of chronic catarrh cases Mucobacter given with an individually-indicated remedy has been very effective.) Six weeks later a dramatic improvement was reported, and he was able to take part in the school choir from which his catarrh had prevented him previously. His father wrote, 'If you were to compare our son's school report for this term with any previous ones you would see why we are so delighted.'

There was a slight relapse a few months later and the symptoms suggested Calc. Carb. 30c, 200c, 1M along with Mucobacter 30c, 200c, 1M. No further trouble was reported.

Difficulty in Passing Exams
A boy of ten had difficulty in passing exams, although apparently of high intelligence.

Past History. Adopted when three weeks old. Much head-banging during dentition. Circumcision at two years. Concussion at three and a half and again at nine years. Nothing known of birth or family history.

On Examination. Healthy, well-built boy. Limitation of movement of the inter-spinal joints of the cervical and upper dorsal region.

Mentals and Generals. Very sympathetic, made many friends, regretted very much if he upset his mother in any way. Got excited easily. Afraid in crowded rooms or in underground trains. Absent-minded, forgot what he has just heard or read or done. Loved sports, very active; very fond of fruit.

Treatment. Gentle manipulation freed the spine. Natrum Mur. covers these mentals and generals; Helleborus was also strongly indicated by this kind of memory defect combined with a history of head injuries. The two remedies are complementary. This type of memory loss is well outside the norm in a boy of apparently high intelligence. Helleborus combined with Natrum Mur. 30c, 200c and 1M on consecutive days was followed by a surprisingly beneficial effect on his examination performance. It had to be repeated some months later following another concussion, and this again was followed by good results. Several months passed without any further trouble and I provided the parents with the prescription named, to be obtained on any future occasions.

Hysteria

A child of nine occasionally fell to the floor breathing heavily with grunting expirations, crying, waving her arms about, always in the presence of someone else, never loses consciousness. This occurs always at home, never at school. She says that she does not know where she is, or whether she is upstairs or downstairs after one of these episodes.

Past History. Very rapid birth. Unusual loss of weight during the first week. No teeth appeared until she was a year old. Father divorced her mother and remarried. Child was staying with her mother and seemed to be well looked after, but at considerable distance from her father. She was very happy any time she saw him.

Concomitants. Fear when she heard splashing of water. Tends to giggle. Says she fears that she is going mad at times. Very interested in religion. Sometimes forgets the immediate past.

Consideration of Treatment. Helleborus covers head injury (rapid birth), loss of memory for the immediate past, insecurity; this is represented in the repertory by 'Homesickness'. Natrum Mur. also has head injury, and experience has shown that it works well in combination with Helleborus in many cases. It covers grief (the loss of her father), and fear of insanity.

Treatment. Helleborus combined with Natrum Mur. was given in the 6c, 9c and 12c potencies on consecutive days. These low potencies were used because there was a possibility that the occurrences might be more severe. This was followed a week later by Lachesis 30c, 200c, 1M, which covers grief, forsaken feeling, fear of water, and hysteria. This was probably too soon after the first prescription, but it was given because the child lived at a considerable distance and it was unlikely that I would be seeing her for nearly two months. I was able to see her six weeks later but the situation was still unsatisfactory.

Lyssin of course covers the fear of water, and is also a head injury remedy. I gave her Lyssin 30c, 200c, 1M on consecutive days; a month later the situation was a little better but still unsatisfactory. I repeated the Lyssin prescription and a month after that it was still really unsatisfactory, although there had been some improvement from the beginning. So I revised the whole case and prescribed Hyoscyamus on the following grounds: it covers head injury, effects of grief, dentition difficult, fear of water, convulsions with consciousness, homesickness, and religious affections. I gave her Hyoscyamus 30c, 200c, 1M on consecutive days and there were no recurrences.

It is difficult to say whether Hyoscyamus should have been given at the start, or whether Helleborus, Lachesis, Natrum Mur. or Lyssin might have prepared the ground. All these cover head injury, which was an outstanding event in this case, and the teaching in homoeopathic practice is to consider physical symptoms to be of prime importance in mental illness.

Menière's Syndrome
A man of seventy-five came to see me on account of Menière's syndrome, which had started five years previously. He had been given nicotinic acid, resulting in freedom for a year, but there was a relapse. He was then put on prochlorperazine, which helped at first but again he relapsed. Nicotinic acid was then tried again, but he had become allergic to it. During the three years before he came to see me he said that he had attacks almost every day lasting for at least eight hours. Attacks consisted of sudden vertigo on rising up from bed in the morning, or in getting up from a seat. He had to do both slowly or else he might fall down – any sudden movement could cause vertigo. There was throbbing in the head generally, and especially in the right ear, which had become completely deaf. His head felt too large for the skull.

Mentals and Generals. Sympathetic to others, disliked sympathy. Could be indifferent to loved ones. Very fond of fish. Generally better living by the seaside. Better for exertion. He had been a keen rugger player, and when free from attacks he felt much better after a brisk walk in the open air. Memory extremely bad, forgot recent events and said he had virtually forgotten everything that had happened during the previous forty years. He could not remember the name of the patient he said I had cured of this disease and who had advised him to come to see me.

Past History. Concussion as a child followed by gingivitis, resulting in the loss of all his teeth.

On Examination. Heavily built. Generally fit. Blood pressure 160/80. Rotation of the neck restricted. Deafness of the right ear.

Treatment. Gentle manipulation of the upper dorsal and cervical intervertebral joints was done, and repeated as required at following consultations. He volunteered later that he felt much better after this treatment. The outstanding events in the past were concussion and its immediate effects. In very early loss of memory, Helleborus is one of the most important remedies (in such cases), and can be combined with other head injury remedies individually indicated.

Helleborus covers head injury, loss of memory for recent events, can be indifferent to loved ones, consolation aggravates, vertigo on rising in the morning or rising from a seat, pulsation in the head, enlarged sensation in the head, pain pressing outwards as if the head was in a vice.

Natrum Mur. covers head injury, better sea air, desires fish, better for exertion, vertigo on rising, worse for motion, pulsation in the head pressing as if the brain was bound up.

Sepia covers head injury, sympathetic, indifferent to loved ones, consolation aggravates, better for sea air, exertion ameliorates, vertigo rising in the morning, rising from sitting, and worse movement of the head, pulsation in the head, pulsation in the ear and deafness.

Calc. Carb. covers head injury, heavy build, sympathetic, consolation aggravates, giddiness in the morning on rising or rising from a seat or moving the head, pulsation in the head and pulsation in the ear, pains of the head as if bound up.

The first prescription was Helleborus Niger 1M combined with Natrum Mur. 1M to be taken daily for four days, followed a week later by Sepia 30c once daily for a week. This was prescribed in a series of numbered powders. The frequency of the dose seemed advisable in view of the frequent and long-lasting attacks.

Two months later he was unable to keep his appointment but wrote to say that he had had only ten attacks in the past month, and that these were of much shorter duration. The prescription was repeated and he kept his next appointment, reporting improvement but still getting attacks. He was then given Helleborus combined with Natrum Mur. 10M, four doses daily without Sepia; this was followed by further improvement, but he still had attacks. The next prescription was Helleborus combined with Calc. Carb. 1M, four doses daily. A month later, he reported that he had had no further attacks. I gave him no more homoeopathic treatment but saw him at monthly intervals for three months and checked any osteopathic lesions, and then discharged him. I had no report of any recurrence during the following two years, after which I lost touch with him.

Footnote. Alumina can cover after-effects of head injury. According to Dr Le Hunt Cooper, aluminium can cause loss of memory and gingivitis. He also believed that Menière's syndrome could be produced, certainly aggravated, by aluminium. This patient had already arranged for the elimination of the use of all cooking and heating utensils made of aluminium, and after questioning him carefully I was reassured that this was being observed.

Spontaneous remission sometimes occurs, making it difficult to assess the value of any kind of treatment. I have treated about a dozen such cases by a combination of homoeopathy, manipulation, and avoidance of the use of aluminium. All were relieved, some relapsed after years of freedom, and all responded to further treatment of this kind.

Migraine (1)

A woman of sixty-four complained of recurrent headaches occurring since the age of thirty-five, following an attack of meningitis treated with penicillin. The headaches were rarely more than two weeks apart, and wet weather or washing the hair could bring one on. At the age of fifty-one she had a fibroid removed. This was followed by considerable bleeding, after which her headaches were worse. A headache consisted of a sore, bruised feeling in the vertex with pressure downwards, and was accompanied by severe pulsation. Talking or lying down aggravated the pain, and the headache then moved to a small spot on the left parieto occipital junction before ceasing. At all stages touch on the head was very painful.

Past History. Concussion at the age of eight. Menstruation was late in commencing and periods lasted for seven days. Individual aspects of menstruation may sometimes be useful in considering constitutional treatment.

On Examination. Generally fit. Slight impairment of movement of the cervical and upper dorsal vertebrae.

Mentals and Generals. An outstanding mental symptom was her intense sympathy to others – she was always concerned for other people, besides her family.

Consideration of Treament. Glonoin and Phosphorus both cover the after-effects of concussion. Head injury, though sometimes difficult to find, is nearly always present in the history of people suffering from migraine. Glonoin and Phosphorus also cover the type of pain in the vertex, and Phosphorus covers pain in a small spot, also pain in the head worse for touch, delayed onset of menstruation and prolonged periods, besides being one of the main remedies for people who are intensely sympathetic to others.

Treatment. After gently freeing the cervical and upper dorsal inter-vertebral joints, I prescribed Phosphorus 30c with Glonoin 30c, three doses every four hours in one day. This was followed by absence of headaches for some weeks, when there was a slight recurrence. A dose of Phosphorus was given and there were no more headaches. Nine months afterwards she suffered a head injury in a car accident, but there was no return of migraine. I saw her a few weeks later and again freed the spine. Following the accident she had become very apprehensive when she saw a red car, reminding her of the car which had caused the accident. For this fear I gave her one dose of Opium 30c, which also covers meningitis. Three months later she complained of being very depressed in the mornings, which through the day gradually left her. For this depression I repeated Phosphorus 30c and Glonoin 30c. No further treatment was required.

Migraine (2)
Man aged forty, for several years suffered from headaches brought on by approach of a thunderstorm, anxiety linked with mental concentration, fluorescent or flickering lights while driving. His headaches always started at about 4 p.m. These headaches were associated with after-images; eyes tested two years earlier and N.A.D., white wine or champagne predisposed to headaches, not other alcohol. Relief was obtained from lying down in the dark, Veganin, and usually much better after sleep.

Concomitants. Rheumatism of shoulders and knees; a marked feature of the knees was that they were very stiff and painful after sitting for any length of time, but relieved by subsequent movement. There was also pain in the joints of the hands and feet, not nearly so severe.

Past History. Forceps were used at birth, and he was slow in walking but was overweight. Recurrent bronchitis until seven, tonsils and adenoids removed, warts on penis and perianal region two years ago which were cauterised. No evidence of venereal disease was claimed.

Family History. Migraine in family, including his mother. His mother's mother had cancer.

On Examination. Tall, slim build, shiny face, some restriction of movement of the neck. Otherwise N.A.D.

Mentals and Generals. Sympathetic to others. Can be indifferent to loved ones at times. Persistent thoughts of unpleasant subjects quite marked. Sensitive to music. Regarding shiny face there are two small rubrics, 'Face, shiny' and 'Face, waxy', which very often contain remedies covering the case. Better at the seaside generally, for which Kent's *Repertory* gives only Medorrhinum. The remedies for aggravation at the seaside sometimes cover 'Better at the seaside', and I take the total list as being influenced by sea air. Natrum Mur., Silica and Carcinosin can be added; Carcinosin sometimes has aggravation on the east coast and amelioration on the south coast, or vice versa. Memory very bad – he forgot what he had just read or decided to do. Desires coffee, drinks about fifteen cups a day. Very fond of fish, salt and fruit. Generally better for physical exertion. Natrum Mur. covers head injury, persistent thought on unpleasant subjects, sympathetic, shiny face, amelioration at the seaside, and a desire for salt, coffee and fruit, better generally for exertion, pain in the occiput extending to the forehead which was characteristic of his headaches. Helleborus covers head injury, indifferent to loved ones and the type of memory defect which was outside the norm at his age. It is complementary to Natrum Mur.

Treatment. I advised discontinuation of food or drink cooked in aluminium, and gave gentle manipulation to free the cervical and upper dorsal intervertebral joints. Natrum Mur. combined with Helleborus 30c, four doses at weekly intervals. At the end of the first month he reported that for the first time he had no headache during the approach of a thunderstorm. He had one headache associated with alcohol. Rheumatic pains had gone from shoulders and knees and there was aggravation of arthritis of the hands and feet. Sac. Lac. was then given, in view of the movement of rheumatic pain from above downwards.

A month later he was free from headaches and the rheumatism had disappeared. Three months later he reported having no further headaches and the craving for coffee had gone. He was generally happier and did not dwell on unpleasant thoughts as formerly. A year after commencing treatment he reported no further headaches, except very occasionally from alcohol.

Schizophrenia

A man of forty-eight was first seen by me with a history of severe depression following the death of his wife two years previously. The diagnosis was made by a leading psychiatrist and he had treatment by drugs and ECT, followed by expert cranial osteopathy without effect.

In addition to the severe depression he had a feeling of great insecurity, concentration was poor and he was very confused. It was difficult for him to make decisions, he was very forgetful, forgetting or misplacing words when speaking or writing, forgot what he had just said or intended to do. He woke up early and found it difficult to get back to sleep, but felt worse generally in the evenings. There was nothing relevant in the family history or in his personal history. I asked him especially if he had experienced any severe head injury but he said that he had no recollection of any. Clinical examination was negative except slight osteoarthritis of the terminal joints of the fourth right finger. Repertorisation indicated consideration of Silica, Graphites and Helleborus Niger.

Treatment. Silica was first given without obvious effect. I made further enquiry about head injury but he still had no recollection of any. Graphites CM was next prescribed, again without any effect, and two months later I saw him for the third time and again went into the past history. This time he suddenly remembered that he had had severe concussion twenty years previously. Helleborus Niger covers loss of memory for the immediate past. It does not usually cover this kind of memory loss at advanced age but his age, and the unusual intensity of the memory loss, certainly pointed to the consideration of Helleborus Niger. It is one of the most valuable remedies for the after-effects of head injury, not only in the recent past.

Helleborus 1M was given one dose daily for three days, and this was followed by considerable improvement. During the next eighteen months he had occasional doses of Helleborus Niger, and within six months was able to take up an appointment entailing international financial banking negotiations. He continued in this work and there was no relapse for another twelve years, at which point I lost contact with him.

Sterility

A woman of thirty-five decided to have a second child, her first one then being four years old. Gynaecological examination had been negative. Temperature charts suggested that ovulation had been taking place.

Family History. N.A.D.

Personal History. Measles at nine months. Concussion at twenty-two, and subsequently she had had three operations to straighten the nasal septum, one before the birth of her child and two afterwards. Recently suffered from vertigo, worse on rising or stooping, and a tendency to fall to the left.

On Examination. Generally fit, but slight scoliosis with limitations to rotation to the neck.

The following homoeopathic remedies were considered. Lachesis covers sympathetic to others, vanishing of thought when speaking, emotional insecurity which she had had from childhood, worse generally before the period, and a scanty period, vertigo with tendency to fall to the left. Lachesis also covers sterility and concussion. Another symptom which is strongly represented in Lachesis is a tendency to dislike clothing, and when convenient this patient used to take all her clothes off in the evening.

Helleborus covers sympathetic to others, vanishing of thought when speaking, emotional insecurity, giddiness on rising and stooping, and a tendency to fall. Helleborus is also one of the main remedies, if not the main one, for the after-effects of concussion.

Silica is also an important remedy both for the after-effects of concussion and sterility; it has emotional insecurity and also the peculiar symptom that she had a very cold nose, hands and feet. This patient also felt much better at the seaside, which is also covered by Silica. Silica covers the giddiness on rising and a tendency to fall sideways.

On the 3rd June I prescribed Lachesis combined with Helleborus 6c, 9c, 12c and 30c on consecutive days. On the 22nd July she reported that the vertigo had been cured. I prescribed a dose of Silica 10M, and saw her again on the 16th October after she had returned from abroad.

In the meantime she had had no return of the vertigo, but had developed a urinary tract infection for which she had been given antibiotics which apparently upset her. I prescribed Nux Vomica 30c, 200c and 1M on consecutive days. In addition to the likelihood of antidoting the after-effects of drugs, Nux Vomica is also an anti-infertility remedy; this treatment was given in November and in the following January she reported being pregnant.

Chapter 29

Lumbago

Osteopathic treatment and homoeopathic treatment have independently cured many cases of lumbago, and they can be combined. One of the homoeopathic remedies which has an excellent record in dealing with lumbago is Rhus Toxicodendron.

Rhus Tox. covers pain worse on beginning to move, including rising from a seat, relief from continued motion, but later there may be recurrence from excess movement; cold wet weather or bathing in the sea causes aggravation, hot baths may provide tremendous relief as in other cases of backache, but this must be avoided as it strongly tends to prevent cure; lukewarm baths can be taken. Rhus Tox. lotion is an additional help, and gentle expert manipulative treatment may be necessary. Rhus Tox. 30c can be given three times a day for four days, then night and morning for three days, after which reassessment can be made. Calc. Fluoride is very similar to Rhus Tox. and fortunately is complementary. It can be given in the same way, and Rhus Tox. lotion can also be used. Individual treatment determined by mental and general symptoms as well as local symptoms may be necessary, as the following case illustrates.

A woman of sixty complained of aching in the lumbosacral region, including both sacro-iliac joints, worse after rising from stooping or rising from bed, and walking on the pavement. Expert osteopathic treatment had been given before I saw her, without any effect.

On Examination. Fairly heavily built. Clinical and X-ray examinations were negative. She had dry lips. Unusually thick fingernails. There were nodosities of the finger joints and callosities on toes.

Mentals and Generals. Menopause. Sympathetic to others. Weeps a great deal. Decisions very difficult. Thinking of complaints aggravates. Scars become painful.

Treatment. Location, sensations, modalities including aggravation from walking, jarring, together with concomitants, thickened nails, callosities on toes, painful scars, dry lips. Mentals and generals indicated Graphites which was given 200c, 1M, 10M on consecutive days, followed by Graphites 6c commencing a week afterwards and repeated at five day intervals for a month. This resulted in complete relief for two years, after which further treatment was required.

Chapter 30

Nasal Catarrh

Sub-acute sinusitis may follow upper respiratory tract infection. In these cases by far the most commonly indicated remedies are, in my experience, Kali Bich., Pulsatilla, or Hydrastis Canadensis. In the majority of cases these are effective in the 200c potency t.i.d. for four days, night and morning for three days. In a number of cases it is very difficult to make the selection, and I have found that these three remedies given in low potency give satisfactory results in most patients.

The prescription is Kali Bich. 6x, Pulsatilla 3c, Hydrastis Canadensis 3x and a 15ml Sig. five drops t.i.d. ex aqua. Alternatively, tablets similarly medicated can be given, two t.i.d. a.c. for three weeks. Should catarrh be very severe, three doses of Mucobacter 30c or 200c given every six hours in one day before commencing the mixture will be found to be effective. It is also advisable to reduce or eliminate milk and cheese from the diet, which may in some cases be absolutely essential. The same treatment can be effective in chronic nasal catarrh, but individually selected remedies are usually necessary, and these can be combined with Mucobacter. If there is a deflected septum, relapses will occur unless this is corrected.

One additional measure is facial massage to stimulate lymphatic drainage. The indication is a doughy feeling inferior to the maxillae on the sides of the nose. The procedure is as follows. Place the fingers very close to the nose both sides, gently press down and draw the fingers, lifting them up and down towards the angle of the jaw. This can be followed by gentle massage of the tissues lying between the posterior and lateral spines of the cervical vertebrae. This should be done for a few minutes, say two or three times a day, by the patient; it is important that massage on the face should be commenced with the fingers right up against the side of the nose, otherwise it may be ineffective. This can of course be carried out by someone other than the patient. This treatment was discovered by a masseuse who carried it out in order to deal with oedema of the face, and found it cured her nasal catarrh.

Chapter 31

Scar Tissue

A girl of eight was admitted to the Royal London Homoeopathic Hospital. This child had been transferred from another hospital at the parent's request, on account of a fairly extensive burn on the chest wall, which had refused to heal. The burn was covered by granulation tissue, and attempts to apply dressings had been abandoned because the patient was terrified at being approached. After a few doses of Graphites 200c the child lost her fear and made a rapid recovery. It could be said that this treatment might have been given just before natural recovery took place. Whether that is the case or not, there is ample evidence supporting the value of Graphites in resolution of granulation tissue and other scars.

Hahnemann's theory of chronic disease has long been the subject of controversy. If an attack of measles was unusually severe, or chronic ill-health followed, Hahnemann regarded this as a flare-up of latent psora, caused by the stimulus of measles. On the other hand, Hering considered that psora was not a single infection, but comprised all epidemic fevers and acute contagious diseases. Tyler agreed with Hering, and I have been impressed greatly by her results of treatment with nosodes of acute infection.

In the treatment of chronic disease, a history of an unusually severe infection, followed by a chronic disease, immediately or after an interval, demands consideration of the appropriate nosode, such as Diphtherinum, Scarlatinum, Morbillinum, Streptococcin, etc. In my experience these unproved nosodes can either be extremely effective or have no effect at all. For this reason it is advisable in the majority of cases to commence treatment with proved remedies, including proved nosodes such as Carcinosin 200c. Professor Paschero claimed that Carcinosin reduced the number of keloid scars caused by plastic surgery.

A woman of twenty-two had been put on the pill at the age of sixteen, as treatment for dysmenorrhoea, until she married when she was twenty, whereafter she was unable to conceive. Folliculinum, which is a synthetic oestrogen, was given on the history of considerable domination by her

181

father, and was followed a week later by Carcinosin 200c. She was pregnant three months later, and shortly after the birth of her first child, was pregnant again. It is possible that Carcinosin dealt with the scarring in the fallopian tube, but of course further proof would be required.

Rubrics covering scar tissue under various headings are to be found throughout Kent's *Repertory*, including, for example, in Generalities under the heading 'Contractions', 'Strictures', 'Stenosis after inflammation', giving forty-six remedies, and Barthel's *Repertory* gives fifty-five. An example of how successful treatment of scar tissue can be achieved by considering mentals, generals, and particulars was given by Dr Stora in a discussion on my first paper 'Homoeopathy and Scar Tissue'.

A man of forty-five suffered from Peyronie's disease. He had incomplete erections making coition impossible, fibrous nodules were present along the urethra. The patient was a nervous, hurried, impatient individual, who sometimes suffered from diarrhoea when emotionally disturbed. He craved sugar and was upset by warmth. The rubrics 'Urethra injury' and 'Urethra knotty' both contain Argentum Nitricum, which obviously covers mentals and generals. A single dose of Argentum Nit. 1M was followed by a complete cure. There was no need to repeat the remedy over several years. This case illustrates the approach to dealing with obvious scars, which can be applied to scars of the skin. (See the rubric and sub-rubric of cicatrices of skin, which may provide part of the clinical picture on which constitutional prescribing for other conditions is based.)

There are unseen scars too, and it is noteworthy that the remedies considered by Hahnemann to be of prime importance in the treatment of chronic disease include Sulphur, Nitric Acid, Thuja and Mercury, all capable of dealing with scar tissue. Unproved nosodes have been prescribed mainly on judgement of the severity of past acute infection, which may be an inaccurate assessment.

A case of duodenal ulcer was handed over to my clinic from another outpatient department. This man had responded well to occasional doses of Graphites 200c, prescribed on mentals, generals and the local indications of relief from warm drinks and lying down. I continued this treatment for several months, then he failed to respond. I felt that it might be unwise to give a higher potency, because in a similar case Graphites CM was prescribed and was shortly followed by perforation. X-rays demonstrated narrowing of the pylorus, and the radiographer expressed his opinion that this was likely to go on to stenosis. On the history of a very severe attack of diphtheria, which was the only childish infection he could remember, I prescribed Diphtherinum 200c, three doses every six hours in one day. This was followed by a great clinical improvement, and a further X-ray was normal. There was no relapse during the following three years.

Unusual severity of an acute infection may presumably determine the degree of after-effects, including scarring, and likewise consideration of the appropriate nosode. Drosera Rotundifolia, in my experience, is the nearest specific for whooping cough. During an epidemic I first gave Drosera 30c t.i.d. for four days, then night and morning for three days, and saw these patients at weekly intervals at the Shepherds Bush Children's Homoeopathic Clinic; the majority were cured within a few weeks. By far the most commonly indicated alternative remedies were Coccus Cacti, the outstanding symptom of which was a paroxysmal cough ending with ropey mucus, clear or white, which hung in long strings from the mouth; and Kali Carb., when there was oedema of the upper eyelids, and sometimes of the cheeks, associated with a typical aggravation at 3 a.m. Sometimes other remedies were needed, including Carcinosin, based on the family history and other symptoms. In cases with a history of severe whooping cough in the past my impression is that Drosera is superior to Pertussin.

Tyler said that the three remedies dealing most successfully with scars have been Graphites, Silica and Drosera; and where tubercular scars are concerned, the greatest of these is Drosera. She also said that she had had a number of cases of tuberculous cervical glands doing well under Drosera, some of them after long treatment here or elsewhere with a great deal of ugly scarring.

What one invariably notices is that the cases that react to this remedy react rapidly, with astonishing improvement in general health. In Drosera cases one notices not only diminution in the size of the gland, but also that the old scars fade away, get free and come to the surface, that discolouration goes, and that when a gland does break down under Drosera, it behaves in a very restrained manner, with small opening and little discharge. It leaves practically nothing to mark what had taken place.

I had the privilege of working as Dr Tyler's clinical assistant and can confirm her remarkable results in tubercular cervical adenitis, as well as in tuberculosis of the mesenteric glands and tuberculosis of bone with discharging sinuses. I remember one case in particular – a child suffering from tuberculosis of the cervical vertebrae – who was cured with Drosera. Such cases are now seen much less frequently, at least in the developed world, and pulmonary tuberculosis has been progressively replaced by carcinoma. Tyler's chapter on Drosera in her *Homoeopathic Drug Pictures* is well worth reading. Drosera has a reputation as a remedy in cases of paranoia. It is interesting that the two remedies in black type in Kent's *Repertory* in the rubric 'Delusions of persecution' are China and Drosera, both scar tissue remedies.

Thiosinaminum, a chemical derived from oil of mustard seed, was introduced into medicine as a remedy for scar tissue, in material doses by mouth or injection. Satisfactory results were claimed but side effects resulted in a trial of Thiosinaminum in potency. References are to be found in Clark's *Dictionary*, Clark's *Prescriber*, Boericke, and Anshult's *New, Old And Forgotten Remedies*. As there are no definite individual indications, I have been prescribing Thiosinaminum alone, or in combination with appropriate remedies, in the thirtieth or two hundredth potency. Over many years I have made more than two hundred prescriptions in these ways, and have come to the conclusion that it is a homoeopathic remedy well worthy of further study. In cases of blockage of the nasolachrymal duct, when scar tissue was suspected, including cases where duct surgery had failed, Dr Douglas Calcott gave Thiosinaminum 3x t.i.d. for two weeks, repeating the course after a two week interval. He told his patients not to expect results until three months after completing these courses.

In more limited experience I have found Natrum Mur. or Silica most often indicated in the treatment of this condition, and successful in the two hundredth potency plussed daily for a week. These are both also scar tissue remedies.

As might be expected, the cases of carpal tunnel syndrome that I have seen have been mainly elderly women, some of whom have developed the condition after a fractured wrist. Constitutionally they almost all worked out to Pulsatilla or Graphites, the Pulsatilla of the menopause. Whether it was a coincidence or not, I have found that these patients were usually sensitive to aluminium, and advised discontinuation of aluminium cooking utensils. It occured to me to give Graphites high, followed by low potencies with the possibility of local effect, and I used a routine Graphites CM followed by a daily dose of Graphites 6c for one month. This usually helped to some extent; combining Thiosinaminum 6c with Graphites 6c was more effective.

A woman of seventy-six had suffered from carpal tunnel syndrome with pain in the neck and upper dorsal region. All pains were worse in the morning and slightly relieved after further movement, but later became worse in the evening. Graphites CM, followed by a nightly dose of Graphites 6c combined with Thiosinaminum 6c was prescribed, with Rhus Tox. lotion to be applied to the painful areas. This helped greatly – she said that she was ninety per cent better, but continued with the Rhus Tox. lotion. She had dispensed with splints, and analgesics were only occasionally used. The prescription had to be repeated on four occasions during the next year, and dealt with any relapse, but the situation was not progressively improving. A feature of past history was that she had recurrent attacks of quinsy over a number of years. This and other symptoms, including its effect on scar tissue, and the fact that it is complementary to Rhus Tox., suggested adding Phytolacca. I prescribed Graphites, Thiosinaminum and Phytolacca 30c to be taken first thing in the morning, mid-afternoon and at bedtime in one day, to be repeated at three-weekly intervals. This resulted in further improvement to the extent that she rarely needed an analgesic, except after driving for a long distance or working hard in the garden. On examination the hands were freely mobile and without pain, but a year later she complained of a slight return of the symptoms. I then prescribed three doses of Morgan Pure, which is complementary to Graphites and Alumina. This resulted in further improvement but had to be repeated six months later, and after that she required no more treatment.

Over the years I have treated about ten such cases, and gave them all Graphites and other post-menopausal remedies such as Lachesis or Sepia when required, as well as remedies associated with amenorrhoea, such as Causticum. I treated one case of a patient who had had two operations and was in considerable pain, and was able to give her great relief by a similar course of treatment.

A woman of eighty-two was in considerable pain from carpal tunnel syndrome, and I obtained a surgical opinion. Operation was advised, but before the operation I prescribed Graphites 30c combined with Thiosinaminum 30c, three times a day for four days, and then night and morning for four days. The pain subsided quite dramatically and the operation was cancelled. Another course was required later, and during the two years following this course there was no relapse.

A man of forty-six complained of tenosynovitis of the flexor tendons of the right wrist, involving the lower third of the forearm, which had developed after an injury. A course of cortisone was given without effect, and it was then put in a plaster of Paris splint again without effect. Surgical treatment was then advised but refused, which was the point at which I first saw him. He noted that the pain was worse on beginning to move in the morning, became slightly easier during the day, and then returned to some extent in the evening. I prescribed Rhus Tox. 30c combined with Thiosinaminum 30c t.i.d. seven days,then b.d. seven days, but this had no effect. On further questioning he remembered that the pain was worse when the weather changed. I gave him a course of Injury Remedy 30c combined with Thiosinaminum 30c and Rhododendron 30c given in the same way, which was successful. He required no more treatment until a year later when there was a slight relapse, and the same prescription proved satisfactory. During the following five years there was no relapse.

One of the most successful uses of Thiosinaminum in my experience is in dealing with post-operative adhesions, either alone or with an individually indicated remedy. As an example of the latter method, a woman of forty-five suffered from what was diagnosed as post-operative adhesions, following hysterectomy six years previously. The symptoms seemed to call clearly for Colocynthis. However, I gave her Thiosinaminum 20c plussed for five days, and then followed up a week later with Colocynthis 3c, twice daily for a week, then night and morning for a week. This was followed by complete relief for two years, when there was a slight recurrence which responded to a similar course of treatment. There has been no recurrence over the next four years. I should add that cases treated by Thiosinaminum alone followed a similar course, the remedy having to be repeated sometimes at long intervals.

A woman of seventy-four complained of constipation associated with sudden painful tenesmus with incomplete evacuations. This started after an operation some years previously to deal with rectal fissure. Mentals, generals and local symptoms were strongly but partially covered by Nitric Acid, which included her allergy to penicillin and her love of driving a car. There were also strong partial indications for Graphites, and a combination of these remedies, both capable of dealing with scar tissue, would probably have been effective. However, in view of the considerable pain and her need to arrange her life to deal with sudden tenesmus, the following prescription was given: Nitric Acid 6c, Graphites 6c, Thiosinaminum 6c, combined t.i.d., a.c. for five nights, then night and morning for five days, then night only for five days. This was very successful, but had to be repeated at increasingly long intervals over the next ten years.

A woman of forty had a laparotomy done on account of abdominal pain. Appendix was normal, a section of the colon was removed as malignancy was suspected but proved negative, and an end-to-end anastomosis was performed. Pain however persisted for three years afterwards until a course of Thiosinaminum 30c one dose daily for a week was prescribed. After five days this had to be discontinued on account of severe pain and weakness of the right shoulder, which had been dislocated on a number of occasions. This cleared up gradually and the abdominal pains were completely cured.

Iris Tenax 30c has had a long clinical reputation of being effective with an attack of appendicitis, but obviously this would be justifiable only if investigation or surgery were not available, and in such circumstances I have occasionally used it. However Dr Jacques Imberechts has found it effective in dealing with scar tissue in the right iliac fossa, and this I have confirmed.

A woman of forty-one complained of mastitis of about ten years duration. There was considerable discomfort and feeling of fullness of the breasts, aggravated by jarring. Sepia 30c was indicated on constitutional grounds, and four doses every twelve hours was prescribed. About a week later a tender swelling developed in the axilla, which resulted in a large and painful carbuncle. Calendula ointment was applied to the carbuncle before and after it discharged. It healed up fairly rapidly, leaving an irregular scarred area about two inches in length, associated with pain from adhesions. Thiosinaminum 30c three times a day for three days, then twice a day for three days was prescribed, resulting in freedom from pain. At the age of twenty this patient had an appendicectomy, and unknown to me, she had suffered from severe sharp pains in the right iliac fossa if she rose quickly up from bed or any other reclining position. Along with relief from pain in the breasts, these pains also disappeared, and there has been no return during the following twenty years.

Vitamin E. Evidence provided by the Shute brothers of Ontario, Canada, said that Alpha Tocopherol could reduce pain in burns when applied locally, and given by mouth besides, reducing scarring. Considering the superior effect of Thiosinaminum in potency, I decided to try potentised Alpha Tocopherol alone, or combined with an individually selected remedy, or with Thiosinaminum. An example of the latter is as follows.

A girl of ten injured her nose through falling from a horse. On examination there was a scar about 2mm wide at the tip of the nose, diminishing in width as it extended upwards for about 30mm. She was seen by a plastic surgeon a few weeks later who reported: 'Examination of the nose shows broadening of the nasal bridge, and there is a definite depression below the nasal bones on the profile view.' He added that nothing could be done at that time, but wished to see the child six weeks later. I prescribed Thiosinaminum 200c combined with Alpha Tocopherol 200c to be given at weekly intervals. The girl was not seen by the plastic surgeon, and during the next four years I gave her an annual course of Thiosinaminum with Alpha Tocopherol 30c, five doses at weekly intervals.

Appendix: Therapeutic Hints

REMEDIES

Aethusa Cynapium 200c is of value to students who 'cannot think' during an examination. A dose in the morning and then, if required, before each part of the examination.

Agaricus Muscarius 200c and Pulsatilla 200c are the two most often indicated remedies for chilblains, covering about two-thirds of cases. Agaricus is worse for cold and has symptoms resembling frost-bite. Pulsatilla is worse in the evening and from exposure to heat.

Alumina 6c, 12c, 30c, 200c, 1M. When repertorising any chronic case, careful note should be made of Alumina symptoms. Alumina is rarely the constitutional remedy, but if there are some characteristic symptoms present, or if the patient suffers from any allergic condition, including eczema and migraine, or from any disease of the alimentary tract, it is advisable for him to avoid eating food prepared in aluminium cooking utensils, or drinks from water heated in an aluminium kettle. It is essential to see that this is carried out completely. Tinfoil used for cooking also contains aluminium, and electric radiators with an aluminium reflector may cause symptoms in sensitive patients. On the whole, it is preferable to use ground coffee beans for making coffee. Many processed foods are prepared in aluminium. It has been suggested that it is impossible to avoid aluminium today. That is so, but the majority of sensitive patients are better off when they avoid it so far as possible, taking a dose of Alumina when symptoms arise. A prescription of the constitutional remedy followed by Alumina given ten to fourteen days later works very well.

Anthracinum 30c or 200c. For boils or carbuncles with much induration, Anthracinum is practically certain to help, without any other indications.

Antimonium Tartaricum 30c, 200c or Antimonium Crudum 30c or 200c are almost specific remedies for impetigo.

Argentum Nitricum 200c can be used for 'examination funk'. This is a well-tested remedy in this respect. It can be combined with Aethusa Cynapium.

Arnica Montana 30c or 200c. This is well known to be the main remedy for surgical shock. The Table on page 194 is a useful guide to pre- and post-operative homoeopathic treatment, combined if necessary with analgesics, and suitably altered individually when required.

Aurum Metallicum 200c, 10M. is a 'pathological' remedy for un-descended testicle, providing the testicle is not ectopic.

Bacillinum and other Tuberculinums are very closely allied to Sulphur in their symptomatology.

Baryta Carb. or Baryta Muriatica are remedies to be considered carefully in old age and when there is arteriosclerosis, but one or other is almost certain to help if a patient looks many years older than his actual age.

Calendula Officinalis is well known for its beneficial effects as an ointment. It is an even more remarkable healing agent given internally in 30c or 200c potency for large wounds, or wounds slow to heal.

Carbo Vegetabilis 3x or 6c, 30c, 200c, is a useful remedy for flatulence in infancy or post-operatively. The indication is relief from eructations. A number of remedies have this, but Carbo Veg. is worth trying when it is definite and the only one. The other two remedies often required in these conditions are Lycopodium, when there is much flatus, and Raphanus when there is 'incarcerated flatus'; the patient is distressed by wind but cannot pass it upwards or downwards. Other remedies, such as Pulsatilla and China, etc., may sometimes be required. In respect of flatulence in infancy it is obviously necessary to see that any feeding mismangement is corrected – these remedies will not be required after this has been achieved in the majority of cases. Aethusa Cynapium is very rarely indicated if correct infant feeding has been established.

Caulophyllum 6c or 30c given one dose daily for three weeks before childbirth has a reputation for making labour quick and easy.

Causticum 200c is the chief remedy for loss of voice from whatever cause. If positive indications for another remedy are absent, it is worth a trial. Causticum is the routine remedy for retention of urine after operation. Rhus Tox. may be required when the bladder muscles have been 'sprained' from distension. After sympathectomy, Hypericum 200c is most likely to be effective. For children who stop growing after a burn, Causticum may be an invaluable remedy.

Chamomilla 6c, half an ounce of tablets, is a useful prescription for teething children. A tablet is given every half hour, up to six doses in any one day, if the child is peevish, irritable, asks for something then throws it away, and is only really at peace when being carried about. It will be effective only if the mental state indicates it.

Chelidonium 1x, 3x, 6c, 30c, is almost a specific remedy when there is pain under the right scapula.

Chininum Arsenicosum 30c is almost a specific remedy for children who get diarrhoea from eggs.

Chloroform 30c, 200c or 1M. When there is a history of severe reaction to chloroform anaesthesia, such as excessive vomiting, and there is liver or gallbladder disease, this may be an invaluable remedy. Children born under chloroform anaesthesia who are liverish may also benefit greatly. It should be considered after caesarian section. In taking a case history it is worthwhile to enquire into any undue effects of anaesthesia. Although it is difficult or even impossible at present to determine the antidote to modern anaesthesia, in which several drugs are employed, older patients may give a clear-cut history of severe reaction to chloroform, ether or nitrous oxide. The appropriate anaesthetic in potency may help greatly in constitutional prescribing.

Cholesterinum 30c, 200c has a beneficial effect on many patients suffering from coronary insufficiency, and may be justified as a prescription when other remedies fail, or if there are no clear-cut indications for another remedy.

Cocculus 30c is the most often indicated remedy for car sickness. A dose should be given before the journey, then as needed. If it is the correct remedy there will be no doubt about it after the first journey.

Coccus Cacti 3x, 30c, 200c is almost a specific remedy for the later stages of whooping cough, or at any stage when there is a paroxysmal cough accompanied by vomiting of thick glairy mucus (like white of egg). It is likely to be useful for any patient with this symptomatology, whatever the cause.

Dioscorea Villosa 6c, 30c, 200c. When a patient suffers from alimentary disorder and obtains relief from bending backwards, this is the first remedy to be considered.

Drosera Rotundifolia 30c or 200c is an almost specific remedy for whooping cough. It can be repeated without harm. As a rule it is probably best given as a single dose and then the effects assessed weekly. Two commonly-indicated remedies to follow are Coccus Cacti or Kali Carb. Indications for the latter are oedema of upper eyelids and an aggravation about 3 a.m. Sometimes the Kali Carb. extreme sensitivity to sudden noises may also be a useful confirmatory symptom.

Euphrasia 30c. When there is marked chemosis associated with conjunctivitis, this points to Euphrasia.

Ferrum Metallicum 30c. For vomiting after tonsillectomy. A dose given after each vomit usually causes rapid improvement.

Ferrum Phosphoricum 2x, Calc. Phos. 3x combined trituration tablets have valuable haematinic properties and do not harm the most sensitive stomach. This prescription can be given in infancy. A useful routine prescription after influenza is Influenza Bacillinum 200c, one dose followed by Ferrum Phos., Calc. Phos. tablets t.i.d., p.c., for a month along with Crataegus Φ, 5 drops ex aqua t.i.d., p.c. for a month.

Gelsemium 3x, 30c, 200c. The mental state which should make one think of Gelsemium is 'feeling miserable'. This, combined with heavy eyes and hot and cold feelings in the back, make the ideal indications for Gelsemium in influenza.

Graphites 200c is almost specific for granulation tissue following burns.

Helleborus 200c, 1M, 10M is a 'pathological' remedy for the after-effects of head injury. It is useful when individual indications are difficult to obtain.

Hepar Sulph. 3x, 30c, 200c is almost a specific remedy for any inflammatory conditions such as boils extremely sensitive to touch and relieved by warmth. Mentals and generals of Hepar Sulph. may or may not be present, but if the patient is in addition irritable and chilly, the prescription can be made with even greater confidence. Sometimes extreme sensitivity to touch is the only definite symptom, and Hepar Sulph. rarely fails then.

Hypericum 6c, 30c, 200c. This remedy is well known for its effects on 'injured nerves' such as in painful abrasions, crushed fingers, and for the after-effects of spinal injury.

Hypericum Oil is an invaluable remedy for bedsores. Hypericum 6c, 12c or 30c internally with hypericum oil has an even more satisfactory effect.

Ignatia 200c, 10M is invaluable to ease the suffering of grief from bereavement. It can be repeated frequently.

Kali Bichromicum 200c and Pulsatilla 200c are the two chief remedies for nasal catarrh continuing after a cold. Kali Bich. has heaviness of the forehead and a stringy discharge. Pulsatilla has a non-stringy bland discharge.

Kali Bromatum 200c may cure acne when apparently indicated remedies fail.

Lachesis 30c, 200c, 1M, 10M should be carefully considered in any post-menopausal disorders.

Lycopodium 200c. When this remedy is suggested from the symptomatology, it is useful to enquire about the kind of anticipation experienced by the Lycopodium patient. If he speaks in public, even though accustomed to doing so, he is typically afraid beforehand, but after commencing to speak, his fears vanish. Lycopodium is a 'pathological' remedy in unresolved pneumonia.

Mancinella 200c. 'Fear of insanity' – probably the main remedy.

Natrum Muriaticum 30c, 200c, or 10M. This remedy should be considered when 'psychic causes of disease' is a prominent feature of the case. An experienced doctor advocated Natrum Mur. for asthma unless there were positive indications for something else. It seems also to be one of the remedies to be considered for patients unduly sensitive to drugs. A short sketch of Natrum Mur. is as follows:
< heat or cold.
< stuffy places; > open air.
< 10 a.m.
Craving for salt.
Easy lachrymation in open air.

Opium CM. When there is a history of fright and the patient experiences fear when the incident is recalled long after.

Phosphorus 200c, 10M is a valuable remedy for pre-operative anticipation, including dental operations.

Pilocarpine 30c is a useful remedy for mumps, t.i.d. 3 days, b.d. 3 days, nocte 3 days.

Pyrogenium 6c, 30c, 200c, 10M. Apart from the symptomatic indications, Pyrogen may be prescribed pathologically when there is a septic focus and toxaemia, bacteraemia or maybe even septicaemia, and when there is either a swinging temperature or a tachycardia out of proportion to the temperature.

Sulphuric Acid 200c. When bruising persists for an unduly long time, whether Arnica has been given or not, Sulphuric Acid is almost always the remedy.

TABLE OF PRE- AND POST-OPERATIVE TREATMENT

| Operation | PRE-OPERATIVE | | | POST-OPERATIVE |
	Evening before	*Morning of Operation*	*Immediately before*	
Hysterectomy	Arnica 30	Arnica 30	Arnica 30	Causticum 30 t.d.s. for 3 days
Gynaecological Repairs	Arnica 30	Arnica 30	Arnica 30	
Dilation and Curettage	Arnica 30	Arnica 30	Arnica 30	Belladonna 30 (III) 6-hourly
Amputation of Breast	Arnica 30	Arnica 30	Arnica 30	Hamamelis 30 (III) 4-hourly
Varicose Veins	Arnica 30	Arnica 30	Arnica 30	Ledum 30 t.d.s. 3 days Hamamelis 30
Appendic-ectomy	Arnica 30	Arnica 30	Arnica 30	Rhus Tox. 30 t.d.s. for 3 days
Partial Gastrectomy	Arnica 30	Arnica 30	Arnica 30	Raphanus 30 t.d.s. for 3 days and s.o. for flatulence
Gallbladder Operations	Arnica 30	Arnica 30	Arnica 30	Lycopodium 30 t.d.s. for 3 days or s.o.s.
Eye Operations	Arnica 30	Arnica 30	Arnica 30	Ledum 30 (III) 4-hourly
Tonsillectomy and Adenoid-ectomy	Arnica 30 (VI) 4-hourly			Rhus Tox. 30 (VI) 4-hourly or s.o.s.
Orthopaedic Operations	Arnica 30	Arnica 30	Arnica 30	Arnica 30
– involving cartilage and periosteum	Ruta 30	Ruta 30	Ruta 30	Ruta 30 (VI) 4-hourly
– including spine	Arnica 30	Arnica 30	Arnica 30	Hypericum 30 (VI) 4-hourly
Mastoidectomy	Arnica 30	Arnica 30	Arnica 30	Arnica 30
Haemorrhoids	Staphysagria 30 4-hourly	Staphysagria 30 4-hourly	Staphysagria 30 4-hourly	Staphysagria 30 4-hourly for 2 or 3 days
	Aesculus 30 4-hourly 2 or 3 days	Aesculus 30 4-hourly	Aesculus 30 4-hourly	Aesculus 30 4-hourly 2 or 3 days
Circumcision	Staphysagria 30 Arnica 30	Staphysagria 30 Arnica 30	Staphysagria 30 Arnica 30	Staphysagria 30 Arnica 30 (VI) 4-hourly

SOME CONDITIONS

1) Appendicitis: when investigation or operation are not available. Iris Tenax 30c repeated as in any acute infection has been extensively found to be satisfactory. Iris Tenax covers post-operative adhesions in the right iliac fossa as well as Thiosinanimum. Give also for tenderness at McBurney's point, frequency according to severity.

2) Asthma attack, better for lying flat on back with legs outstretched. Give Psorinum in the attack.

3) Aware of heart. Spigelia 30c or 200c.

4) Bruising persisting. Consider Sulphuric Acid 200c, especially if there is discolouration.

5) Carsickness. See rubrics for 'Nausea Riding in a Carriage', and 'Vomiting Riding in a Carriage'. Treat on constitutional symptoms.

6) Cracked thumbs. Nitric Acid 6c (20 minims), Petroleum 6c (20 minims) in Calendula ointment.

7) Despair of recovery (mainly in acute illness). Consider Psorinum.

8) Diarrhoea after penicillin. Nitric Acid is almost a specific.

9) Emotional insecurity. See rubrics on 'Homesickness' in the repertories.

10) Fastidiousness. Consider Alumina, Anacardium, Arsenicum Alb., Carcinosin, Conium, Graphites, Nux Vomica, Phosphorus, Platina, Pulsatilla, Sepia.

11) Ingrown toenail. Magnetic Polus Australis 200c, 3 doses every twelve hours.

12) Nosebleed. Apart from other measures, Millefolium 200c or 10M. If these are not available, consider Ferrum Phos. 30c or 200c.

13) Osteoarthritis of feet. Manganum 12x alternating with Hecla Lava 12x daily for a month. May also be useful at other sites.

14) Osteoarthritis of finger or toe joints. Consider Caulophyllum 6c, especially in post-menopausal women. Can be combined with the constitutional remedy.

15) Pain in the veins. Pulsatilla 3x, Fluoric Acid 3x, Hamamelis 3x.

16) Post-operative flatulent distension. (i) Better for eructation almost always responds to Carbo Veg. 30c or 200c, six doses, half- to two-hourly. (ii) Better for passing flatus responds to Lycopodium 30c or 200c, six doses, half- to two-hourly. (iii) Not relieved by eructation or flatus – almost always responds to Phytolacca 30c, six doses, half- to two-hourly, or Pulsatilla in the same dosage.

17) Premenstrual oedema. Apocynum 30c daily for a few days.

18) Radiation. Phosphorus is one of the best antidotes. Phosphorus is also useful after X-rays, although Fluoric Acid is better. Consider X-ray 30c or 200c intercurrently with Radium Bromide 30c or 200c. Also, Cadmium 100c as well as Phosphorus 100c are antidotes to radium burns (Grimmer).

19) Sprained ankle. Arnica 30c if seen on day of accident, followed by Rhus Tox. 30c twice daily for three days; or Rhus Tox from the start if seen on the second day. If it is judged that there is much tearing of the attachment or Achilles tendon, Ruta can be given instead of Rhus Tox. In the same way, Ledum 30c has been extensively used at all stages, and could be given if exact.

20) Tenderness over liver area (chronic, or else related to an acute condition such as influenza). Chelidonium mother tincture five drops in water twice daily can be given with a constitutional remedy, including Carcinosin. It can also be given in repeated doses of Gelsemium in influenza, where Gelsemium 200c is given two-hourly. Carduus Marianus mother tincture seems to act more effectively when tenderness is mainly found on the left side of the liver. It can be given in the same way as Chelidonium mother tincture, along with constitutional or acute remedies. On the whole, Chelidonium seems more often indicated, or else should be preferred if the situation is not clear.

21) Undescended testicle in Down's syndrome. Aurum Met. 200c.

22) Voice loss. Three common remedies. If no clear indications, consider Causticum. Following a cold, consider Rhus if the modalities are better for use of voice and in warmth. Consider Phosphorus if the cords are coated with mucus which must be coughed up.

23) Weakness and restlessness, including sometimes even going from one bed to another. Consider Arsenicum Alb.

24) Weakness apparently out of proportion to severity of illness, with or without restlessness. Consider Arsenicum Alb.

SOME THERAPEUTIC HINTS IN CHILDREN

Note: The indicated potencies are merely suggestions.

1) For the excessively obstinate child, Tub. Bov. 30c or 200c is most often indicated.
2) A craving for affection in children very often indicates Pulsatilla, Phosphorus and Calc. Phos. Pulsatilla accepts affection, Phosphorus accepts and returns it. Calc. Phos. is much less often required.
3) For the child who never looks clean or who is deliberately dirty in his habits, Sulphur 200c is nearly always the remedy.
4) For mental tension not always apparent on admission but realised after a period of observation, Dysentery Co. 200c is the most likely remedy.
5) For pre-operative anticipation Phosphorus 200c can be given in conjunction with Arnica or other pre-operative medication.
6) For homesickness think of Capsicum 200c first, but there are many other remedies.
7) For post-operative vomiting induced by and only occurring after eating, Ferrum Metallicum 30c is nearly always the remedy.
8) For the child who makes a pretence of weeping, but without tears, Staphysagria 30c or 200c is almost certainly the remedy.
9) When a 'blanket of chemotherapy' is apparently indicated, try Pyrogen 200c, a few doses pre- and post-operatively, and reserve chemotherapy to be used later if really required, unless there is overwhelming infection.
10) For otitis media, Hepar Sulph. 200c should be given in the absence of clear-cut indications for another remedy.
11) Nine out of ten cases of infective hepatitis in children need Phosphorus.
12) Senna 6c given half-hourly to two-hourly for a few doses has a specific effect on ketosis associated with febrile disturbance in children, and can be given as a pathological remedy as well as the individual prescription.

Index of Remedies

Cardiovascular Problems in Practice, Dr Roger Blackwood, 1986. A practical guide to the management of the cardiological emergencies and problems that form part of the daily work of the non-specialist doctor.   0906584167

Disorders of Cardiac Rate, Rhythm and Conduction, Dr Hamish Watson, 1984. Detailed guidance on the use of the ECG in the diagnosis and management of the cardiac patient. Written for the general practitioner, hospital doctor and cardiac nurse.   0906584108

Handbook for Care, Muriel Flack, SRN and Margaret Johnston, RGN, 1986. A practical textbook for care assistants/nursing auxiliaries working in the community, in hospital or in the residential care sector.   0906584132

Herbal Medicine, Dr. R. F. Weiss, 1988. The leading textbook of medical herbalism. A systematic study of plant drugs within a framework of clinical diagnoses, with a wealth of suggested prescriptions.   0906584191

Hysterectomy and Vaginal Repair, Sally Haslett, SRN and Molly Jennings, MCSP, 1988. For the patient – explains these operations and how to prepare for them. Advice on what to do afterwards for a trouble-free return to normal life.   090658423X

Nursing for Continence, Christine Norton, SRN, 1986. The definitive text on the nursing care of the incontinent patient.   0906584159

Lymphoedema: Advice on Treatment, Dr Claud Regnard, Caroline Badger, SRN and Dr Peter Mortimer, 1988. For the patient – explains what lymphoedema is and provides a daily management plan that can be followed at home.   0906584248

Oral Morphine in Advanced Cancer (2nd Edition), Dr Roger Twycross and Dr Sylvia Lack, 1989. Explains in detail how to use oral morphine most effectively in the management of cancer pain.   0906584272

Oral Morphine: Information for Patients, Families and Friends, Dr Robert Twycross and Dr Sylvia Lack, 1988. Offers answers to questions frequently asked by cancer patients when advised to start morphine therapy.
0906584221

Surgery and Your Heart, Mr Donald Ross and Barbara Hyams, 1982. Colour-illustrated booklet for patients facing, or who have recently had, heart surgery.
0906584078

What Shall I Do? Questions and Answers in Cardiology, Dr Roger Blackwood and Dr Bev Daily, 1988. Questions from a GP and answers from a cardiologist on the cardiological queries that can be expected to arise in general practice.
0906584205

The Beaconsfield Homoeopathic Library

Classical Homoeopathy, Dr Margery Blackie, 1986. The complete teaching legacy of one of the most important homoeopaths of our time. 0906584140

Everyday Homoeopathy, Dr David Gemmell, 1987. A practical handbook for using homoeopathy in the context of one's own personal and family health care, using readily available remedies. 0906584183

Homoeopathic Prescribing, Dr Noel Pratt, revised 1985. A compact reference book covering 161 common complaints and disorders, with guidance on the choice of the appropriate remedy. 0906584035

Homoeopathy as Art and Science, Dr Elizabeth Wright Hubbard, 1989. The selected writings of one of the foremost modern homoeopaths.

0906584264

Homoeopathy in Practice, Dr Douglas Borland, reprinted 1988 with Symptom Index. Detailed guidance on the observation of symptoms and the choice of remedies. 090658406X

Insights into Homoeopathy, Dr Frank Bodman, 1989. Homoeopathic approaches to common problems in general medicine and psychiatry.

0906584280

Introduction to Homoeopathic Medicine (2nd Edition), Dr Hamish Boyd, 1989. A formal introductory text, written in categories that are familiar to the medical practitioner. 0906584213

Materia Medica of New Homoeopathic Remedies, Dr. O. A. Julian, paperback edition 1984. Full clinical coverage of 106 new homoeopathic remedies, for use in conjunction with the classical materia medicas. 0906584116

Studies of Homoeopathic Remedies, Dr Douglas Gibson, 1987. Detailed clinical studies of 100 major remedies. Well-known for the uniquely wide range of insights brought to bear on each remedy. 0906584175

Tutorials on Homoeopathy, Dr Donald Foubister, 1989. Detailed studies on a wide range of conditions and remedies. 0906584256

– NOTES –

– NOTES –

– NOTES –

– NOTES –

– NOTES –

– NOTES –

– NOTES –

– NOTES –